PROFESSIONAL ETHICS
IN HEALTH CARE SERVICES

PROFESSIONAL ETHICS IN HEALTH CARE SERVICES

Edited by
Eugene Kelly

The Long Island Philosophical Society

UNIVERSITY
PRESS OF
AMERICA

Lanham • New York • London

Copyright © 1988 by

University Press of America,® Inc.

4720 Boston Way
Lanham, MD 20706

3 Henrietta Street
London WC2E 8LU England

Printed in the United States of America

British Cataloging in Publication Information Available

Co-published by arrangement with The Long Island Philosophical Society

Library of Congress Cataloging-in-Publication Data

Professional ethics in health care services / edited by Eugene Kelly. p. cm.
Papers were presented at the Conference on Professional Ethics in Health Care Services, held on
Mar. 21, 1987 at the New York Chiropractic College on Long Island, sponsored by the Long
Island Philosophical Society.
1. Medical personnel—Professional ethics—Congresses. 2. Healers—Professional
ethics—Congresses. I. Kelly, Eugene, 1941–   . II. Conference on Professional Ethics in Health
Care Serivces (1987 : New York Chiropractic College) III. Long Island Philosophical Society.
[DNLM: 1. Delivery of Health Care—congresses. 2. Ethics,
Medical—congresses. W 50 P9634 1987]
R724.P73   1988   174'.2—dc 19   DNLM/DLC for Library of Congress   88–27691 CIP
ISBN 0–8191–7211–1 (pbk. : alk. paper)
ISBN 0–8191–7210–3 (alk. paper)

All University Press of America books are produced on acid-free paper.
The paper used in this publication meets the minimum requirements of
American National Standard for Information Sciences—Permanence of Paper
for Printed Library Materials, ANSI Z39.48–1984.

TABLE OF CONTENTS

PREFACE

The papers contained in this volume were presented at a conference that unique is in both its content and in the professional interactions it produced. The Conference on Professional Ethics in Health Care Services was held on March 21, 1987 at the New York Chiropractic College on Long Island. The Long Island Philosophical Society took on its sponsorship after receiving the original impulse to such a conference from the President of New York Chiropractic College, Dr. Ernest G. Napolitano. Dr. Napolitano met in 1984 with members of the Executive Committee of the Society to discuss his plans for integrating studies in the humanities, and especially in ethics, in the program of study of all chiropractors in this country. The conference he proposed was intended to bring together philosophers specializing in ethical analysis and members of the non-allopathic health care professions to examine the ethical issues that arise in these professions, at least some of which are relatively new to the American scene.

The generous funding provided by Dr. Napolitano, and the invitation to hold the conference at the College's new facilities in Old Brookville led to the Society's issuing a nationwide call for papers. The response we received was highly gratifying, and plans were made to hold the conference in the fall of 1985. Dr. Napolitano's sudden death in June, 1985 caused a postponement that might have become permanent, had it not been for two developments: the continuing support of the new President of New York Chiropractic College, Dr. Neil Stern, and the receipt of a grant from the New York Council for the Humanities. These new funds permitted the Society to extend its invitation to the philosopher Dr. Michael Bayles of Florida State University. His keynote address provided a unifying vision of the tasks of ethical analysis which engaged our invited speakers in each of their health care professions.

The degree of consultation among the speakers and their commentators prior to the conference was unusual for any similar event that I have worked on in the past, and perhaps indicates both the level of mutual engagement in the task of ethical analysis on the part of the moral philosophers and health care representatives, and the ground-breaking content of the program itself. Indeed, the level of discussion generated during the conference itself, and the concern for sharing divergent insights was gratifying to all the persons who made the conference possible. We are confident that many of the essays in the present volume will find their place in the literature as constituting significant contributions to the field of professional ethics. I would like now to mention the names of those who contributed their time and expertise in philosophy and health care to the realization of the conference itself, and to the present volume of papers that come out of it.

The work of reading and selecting among papers sent to us was undertaken by a committee consisting of members of departments of philosophy of Long Island colleges: Dr. Harold Allen, Adelphi University, Dr. Maureen Feder - Marcus, State University of New York at Old Westbury, Dr. Philip Pecorino, Queensborough Community College, and Dr. Evelyn Shirk, Hofstra University. Special thanks are owing to Dr. Luis E. Navia, New York Institute of Technology, who contributed much time to the staging of the conference itself. Assistance in publicizing the conference was given by the Philosophy Documentation Center in Bowling Green, Ohio; assistance in reaching members of the nursing profession was given by Janet Palombo of the New York State Nurses' Association and by Professor Elsie Bandman of the Department of Nursing of Hunter College, New York. Janet Groce of the New York Council for the Humanities was especially helpful to Dr. Pecorino, who first drafted the grant proposal, and to me, as we worked against deadlines to complete it for presentation to the Council. Many hours of assistance were contributed to the book production process by Charles Kirst and Stanley Silverman of the New York Institute of Technology, who are past masters of the computer software and hardware technology that are utilized today in word-processing and in the printing of near-typeset quality text. And finally, the Executive Committee of the Long Island Philosophical Society wishes to extend its thanks to Beatrice and Oscar Bekoff, who are longtime friends and generous supporters of the Society.

Eugene Kelly
Spring 1988

PROFESSIONAL ETHICS IN HEALTH CARE SERVICES

PROFESSIONAL DISOBEDIENCE IN NURSING: THE MORAL DUTY TO DISOBEY

By Jane Brody, Ph.D.
Molloy College

Introduction

When most nurses think about ethical problems, they think in terms of dilemmas -- difficult choices between two morally desirable but mutually exclusive courses of action. However, many nurses are not troubled because they are faced with two options both which are equally supported by moral principles. Many nurses are troubled because either the option that they have already chosen as the ethical course of action is not within their capacity to implement or they know that they are not meeting their ethical responsibilities to the patient but do not know how to effect a change that would rectify this.

Nurses, from their strategic position within the health care field, can see the quality of patient care suffer as a result of incompetent health professionals, inflexible institutional policies, and an overburdened health delivery system that cannot meet the demands made upon it. Those nurses who recognize the dehumanization and debasement of patient care are disturbed by their acquiescence and participation in the process but often feel incapable of effecting changes to improve the situation.

The inability of nurses to provide the level of care that they desire strikes at the very foundation of nursing practice and can lead to what various authors call professional disillusionment, reality shock, and moral distress (Corwin, 1961; Jameton, 1984; Kramer, 1974). All three problems relate to the sense of frustration, sadness, and anger that nurses feel about their practice. Of the three, moral distress emphasizes the ethical component of the situation. Moral distress occurs when the nurse knows the right thing to do, "but institutional constraints make it nearly impossible to pursue the right course of action" (Jameton, 1984, p. 6).

3

Nurses are expected to follow prescriptions and implement decisions in which they had little or no voice while maintaining a sense of moral responsibility for their actions and the consequences of their actions. However, when the perception of choice, autonomy, and participation in decision making is low, many people feel less morally responsible for the outcome of their actions (Gomperz, 1939; Gilligan, 1982). Because of the nature of their practice, which involves the welfare of others, nurses must feel responsible for the outcome of their actions even when they possess few decision-making powers.

Although specific ethical dilemmas -- such as participation in abortion -- need to be addressed by the nursing profession, the two major ethical issues in nursing identified by Curtin, editor of *Nursing Management*, are the "usurpation of the legitimate authority of the nurse vis-a-vis nursing decisions regarding nursing care" and dilemmas which arise from institutional policies and physician orders (Curtin, 1978, p. 8).

The concept of professional disobedience addresses these issues of authority and autonomy in nursing practice directly. Abrams, (1980) who developed the term "professional disobedience," defined it as the refusal of nurses to carry out immoral or unsafe orders from authorities higher in the health care hierarchy. Prior to the discussion about professional disobedience, an overview of autonomy and authority in nursing practice will be presented to provide a framework for the moral duty to disobey.

Perspectives on Nursing and Health Care

Nursing has three complementary aspects of practice-dependent, independent, and interdependent (Flaherty, 1980). Nurses must differentiate and demarcate these three components in order to clarify their ethical responsibilities and to provide quality care to patients within the bureaucratic settings where they practice.

Aroskar (1982) used the term "mindset" to describe four patterns for perceiving health care that influence nursing practice. These different "mindsets" tend to emphasize either the dependent aspects of nursing practice or the independent/interdependent aspects of nursing practice. These four "mindsets" are: health care viewed as medical cases; health care viewed as a commodity provided by the hospital; health care as the patient's right -- this is the patient advocacy position; and health care viewed as cooperative effort to promote the patient's well-being. Each of these four "mindsets" and their ethical implications for nursing practice will be explored as framework for understanding professional disobedience.

The first "mindset" is health care viewed as medical cases. This "mindset" subordinates nursing entirely to medicine and encourages "blame avoidance behaviors" by nurses who often fail to recognize and to assume responsibility for their practice because of their feelings of powerlessness and dependency in the traditional nurse/physician relationship (Stanley, 1978, 1140). The rationale for nursing actions is "the doctor ordered it". This "mindset" also contains a sexist viewpoint that the proper role for nurses, ninety-five percent of whom are women, is to be passive and obedient to the male medical hierarchy.

The traditional relationship between the doctor and the nurse was once one of dominance by the physician and deference and obedience by the nurse. At the turn of the century the *American Journal of Nursing* published an article which stated, "Obedience is one of the abiding virtues. From the beginning to the very end of a nurse's career it must be maintained, and no nurse is exempt..." (Perry, 1906).

This historical perspective has changed. There is some recognition that the authority of others over nursing is limited to particular areas of practice. The obedience and duty of nurses is circumscribed.

Physicians have the authority in medical diagnosis and therapy because of their expertise based on extensive education and training in those fields. Those areas of nursing practice which overlap with medical diagnosis and treatment will be affected by the physician's authority. However, no area of nursing practice is truly dependent. Legal precedent has established the necessity of nurses challenging the treatment of patients by physicians when it falls beneath community based standards (Walker, 1983).

Physicians had come to believe that they have the sole professional relationship with the patient and all others who wish to work with the patient require their approval. This attitude is still subtly expressed in the expression, "Mr. Jones is Dr. Smith's patient", rather than "Dr. Smith is Mr. Jones's physician".

"The physician regards other health care professionals as mainly serving him in his so-called captain of the ship role rather than the whole team working side by side serving the patient" (Kalisch & Kalisch, 1977, p. 52). Physicians have been slow to recognize their dependence on other health care professionals or the important contributions to the patient's welfare made by these other professionals without physician participation. The fact that much of "nursing care goes on without either the consultation or presence of the doctor" is still not recognized (Aroskar, 1980, p. 28).

The second "mindset" is health care viewed as a commodity provided by the hospital. The nurse with this "mindset" feels primary responsibility to the hospital and the rationale for nursing actions is the claim "I'm just following hospital policy."

The hospital employment setting with groups of nurses sharing care for a group of patients does not foster individual responsibility. The hierarchial nature of most institutions further remove accountability from the patient/nurse interaction (Labelle, 1978). Institutional policies and goals may not only frustrate nurses who attempt to practice according to the basic moral principles of the system, but in some cases the policies and goals may contribute to the moral blindness and unwillingness to think in terms of ethical concerns (Wakins, 1985).

Roberts (1986a, 1986b), in a current series of articles in the *American Journal of Nursing*, identifies several "Games Nurses Play" which perpetuate irresponsibility through actions which "never take a chance, never offer a suggestion, and by no means make a decision." Other nurses strive to be models of cooperation and congeniality partially based on their socialization that these are the proper female

6

behaviors. Passing problems to higher authorities and focusing on meaningless details so that all action grinds to a halt are two other games which used to avoid responsibility (Roberts, 1986b).

Both of the above two "mindsets" -- health care viewed as medical cases and health care viewed as a commodity provided by the hospital -- curtail nurses' autonomy and their development as moral professionals. Nurses with these "mindsets" are satisfied to remain in a subordinate position and blindly follow the orders of anyone with authority within the health care hierarchy. In doing so, they fail to assume responsibility for their practice (Lieberman, 1973, p. 39).

These "mindsets" reinforce the dependent aspects of nursing practice while ignoring the independent. Although a small portion of nursing practice is dependent on authority of others, the attitude of dependence becomes a problem when nurses do not control the aspects of their practice which could and should be independent.

Many nurses have been reluctant to recognize the independent nature of their practice. "A lack of knowledge and assertiveness, a fear of failure, a fear of assuming responsibility, and a fear to be held accountable for their actions foster the development and maintenance of passive dependence" (Ritter, Crulcich, & McEntegart, 1981, p. 7).

The unwillingness of many nurses to assume responsibility for decision making and the lack of support for nurses who try to increase their level of autonomy have limited nursing's efforts to achieve parity in the health care system. Many nurses have been too passive professionally and have seemed to be more comfortable responding to others than initiating action. For the practice of nursing to be considered ethical, nurses must accept accountability for their actions directly to the patient rather than shifting their accountability to other health care authorities.

The third "mindset" is health care viewed as the patient's right. Nurses with this "mindset" view themselves as patient advocates. This perception of a nurse's responsibility to the patient developed in the late 1960's and early 1970's with the rise of con-

7

sumerism and feminism, and the post-Watergate distrust of authority. As the previously unlimited authority of the physician shrank, the power of the patients grew. The advent of advocacy by the nurses was partly in recognition of the increasing power of patients as embodied in their new found rights-- privacy, confidentiality, autonomy, and respect. The advocacy role focuses almost entirely on the patient's right to autonomy. It assumes that autonomy is the highest patient welfare.

The present American Nurses' Association (ANA) code of ethics which was revised in the 1970's reflects this changing perception of the nurse.s moral responsibilities in statements such as "the nurse's primary commitment is to the client's care and safety. Hence, in the role of the client advocate, the nurse must be alert to take appropriate action regarding any instances of incompetent, unethical, or illegal practice(s) by any member of the health care team or the health system itself, or any action on the part of others that is prejudicial to the client's best in- terest"(ANA, 1976, p. 3).

Nurses often confuse the advocacy role with defending or rescuing the client which can foster patient dependency and low self-esteem. "We should and can become patients' advocates in the truest sense, the intermediaries for the befuddled civilian who is thrust into the maze of an alien world -- the American health care system" (Christy, 1973). There is an underlying bias that the nurse is always working in the patient's best interest while other health professionals are not. Nurses are often quick to point out the failures of the system, but overlook the part that nurses themselves play in dehumanizing patient care.

The role of the patient advocate is to inform the patient and then sit back and let the patient decide for himself or herself without coercion, threat, or persuasion. The values and wishes of the patient become the deciding factors in determining nursing actions. Kohnke (1982, p. 82) in her book, *Advocacy: Risks and Reality,* states, "Judgment is not part of the role of the advocate; the advocate's duty is only to insure the right of free will or free choice".

After the role of information giver is over, the nurse becomes a bystander in the whole decision-making process of the patient. However, this disinterested position is contrary to the fiduciary relationship between the nurse and the patient which is based on the assumption that the nurse is concerned for the patient's welfare.

In "mindsets" where doctor, hospital, or patient act as the source for the moral legitimacy of nursing, nurses have lost touch with their own professional moral responsibilities and autonomy of practice. As physicians, hospital administrators, and patients use nurses to provide what they have determined is acceptable nursing care, nurses become primarily means to the ends of others (Aroskar, 1982, p. 28). Nurses are not independent practitioners, but rather, dependent figures whose actions are prescribed by the physician, hospital or patient.

Some nurses would prefer to avoid actively participating in decisionmaking under the mistaken belief that this lack of participation removes from them any moral responsibility for their actions that are a result of the decision. They fail to see that they have already made a choice -- a choice not to choose -- and that they cannot escape moral responsibility for their own practice.

Although there are acknowledged duties that nurses have to the physician and the hospital, legally and ethically, because of the dependent nature of a small portion of their practice and their status as employees of an institution, the fundamental duty of the nurse is to the patient. Neither the institutional settings nor the authorities within it remove this responsibility for nursing practice from nurses. Nurses cannot hide behind bureaucratic red tape and other health care professionals. Although to a large extent what a nurse can do is limited by the employing agency, other health care workers in that agency, and the consumer of health care, the largest determining factors are the nursing profession and the nurse (Nuckolls, 1974, p. 629). In the complex situations where health care is given, the moral responsibility for controlling nursing practice must rest with the nursing profession.

Aroskar's (1982) fourth "mindset" is health care viewed as a cooperative effort to promote well-being. The doctor, the patient, the administrator, and the nurse are all considered equal partners working toward the common goal of patient well-being. In this fourth "mindset", "the client is still the focus of care delivery, but the process implies all participants are individually respected for their contributions... Both providers and clients have rights and responsibilities..." (Aroskar, 1982, p. 29). However, before the interdependency of health professionals can occur, there must be recognition of the independent aspects of nursing practice. "Interdependence is based on the autonomy of each profession" (Ritter, Crulcich, McEntegart, 1981, p. 12). However, this interdependent form of practice is blocked because the freedom and the ability of the nurse to act on the patient's behalf independently of other health care professionals is still questioned. Thus autonomy is a key moral issue in nursing practice.

"Autonomy implies independence, responsibility, accountability, self-determination, and self-regulation" (Dachelet & Sullivan, 1979, p. 15). Autonomy is a troublesome ethical issue for nurses who "in contrast with physicians and patients, ... are usually not considered primary decisionmakers" (Aroskar & Veatch, 1977, p. 23).

The autonomy that nurses seek is not the freedom to do as they please at all times. Nurses seek work-related autonomy -- the ability to practice according to the standards of the nursing profession in order to insure the quality of care provided (Engel, 1970). "Professional autonomy is justified ... not as a symbol of, nor reward for catching the coveted, if tarnished brass ring of professionalism ... (It is justified) on the basis of enabling our greatest contribution to the public welfare (Styles, 1982, p. 97).

Nurses do still have autonomy. They can exercise their autonomy in many different ways. Professional disobedience is just one method to clarify the independent portions of nursing practice and to help safeguard the quality of care patients receive. Professional disobedience supports the independent

actions of nurses so they can then work inter-
dependently with other health care providers.

Professional Disobedience

Professional disobedience is not "an assertion of
freedom or a claim to rights. It is an acknowl-
edgment of a new but undeniable obligation" (Walzer,
1967, p. 163). Professional disobedience is not the
outgrowth of newly acquired rights to autonomy for
nurses. It is the response to increased awareness of
nursing's responsibility and ability to insure the
quality of patient care.

Disobedience is usually a collective activity.
"Throughout history, when men have disobeyed or
rebelled, they have done so, by and large, as members
or representatives of a group, and they have claimed,
not merely that they are free to disobey, but that
they are obligated to do so" (Walzer, 1967, p. 163).

Duties begin with membership in a group,
especially when it is a willful membership. Obligations are incurred and felt through social interaction
(Walzer, 1967). When people choose to become
nurses, they enter a profession which has established
standards of ethical conduct. The professional
collective provides the forum for debate and resolution of practice issues and the setting of standards
for practice and evaluation. When nurses do not meet
this established professional level of conduct, they
have breached their duty as nurses.

In professional disobedience, a nurse chooses not
to conform to the orders of superiors because the
professional standards developed by the nursing
community for her public role as nurse are being
compromised (Abrams, 1980). Professional disobedience is tied to the duties a nurse has in her
public role and the shared standards of the profession
are used to justify its use.

Patient care requires the collaborative efforts of
many health professionals. Nurses want to be
participants in the overall health care delivery system,
but they still want control over their aspect of it,
nursing practice. Nurses have a duty to their
patients to maintain the quality of their practice

11

when the hospital system interferes. Professional disobedience may be required to limit the interference into nursing practice which can imperil the quality of patient care.

The term "professional disobedience" developed by Abrams (1980) originally meant the refusal of nurses to carry out an immoral or unsafe order from authorities higher in the health care hierarchy. This refusal is based on the maxim "Do no harm". This is the moral principle of nonmaleficence which is negative duty, the obligation not to cause iatrogenic illness and injury. Because of the patient's right to safe ethical care, the nurse is obligated to challenge orders which would jeopardize that care. The nurse's obligation to follow hospital policies or physician's orders arises from the assumption that in doing so, the nurse is acting in the patient's best interests (Muyskens, 1982, p. 56). However, when this assumption is no longer valid -- that is when hospital policies or physician's orders are not in the patient's best interest -- the nurse must disobey.

In order to address the issues of moral distress and the dehumanization of patient care, the definition of professional disobedience has been enlarged to include the acceptance of responsibility for initiating changes in the hospital setting which will improve patient care. This definition of professional disobedience is derived from the positive duty to do good, benevolence.

The expanded scope of action for professional disobedience is more compatible with Muyskens' (1982) position that nurses are not victims (or impotent bystanders) in the debasement of health care, but accomplices. Parson (1986, p. 275) states, "if nurses are to create new standards that complement rather than conflict with their own views of what is acceptable professional practice, they must confront norms of employing institutions that block the attainment of professional goals." Professional disobedience is a form of confrontation.

Abrams (1980) discusses individual action that nurses can pursue when moral distress occurs. When nurses are expected or ordered by their superiors or employers to perform nursing functions which conflict with basic ethical premises of the profession (nonmaleficence and beneficence), they should refuse to carry out the order. Such refusal should be done openly so as to shed light on the problem and help prevent its reoccurrence.

The guidelines developed by Abrams (1980) for profession disobedience are:

1. Professional non-compliance must be undertaken only in situations where the ethical breach is large. It should never be undertaken lightly and it should never become a common occurrence.
2. Normal avenues for correction of the problem should have been tried prior to becoming professionally non-compliant. Professional disobedience is an action of last resort when other established methods of solving the problem have failed.
3. Professional non-compliance should never occur when it could break a major ethical principle. For example, if being disobedient could cause harm to the patient, it is not justifiable.
4. To be considered professional non-compliance-- rather than a personal moral action -- the ethical principle that the non-compliance addresses must be one commonly shared by the system in which the nurse is employed. A nurse may refuse to assist with abortions, but that is a personal decision, not professional disobedience. Professional disobedience adheres to the standards of nursing practice established by nursing as a whole.

Disobedience must be morally justifiable. Those who disobey must be willing to act in public, explain their actions, and take responsibility for the consequences. However, these steps in themselves do not legitimate the disobedience, only the acknowledged obligation to fulfill explicit commitments and maintain established communal principles can provide adequate justification. (Walzer, 1967, pp. 170-173).

Margretta Styles, president of the American Nursing Association, states that it is the collective of nursing colleagues which not only provides the standards for nursing, but also stands "behind the nurse, who ... has to push against the constraints of the profession or the social context to push out the boundaries of practice" to insure and enhance the quality of nursing care (Styles, 1982, pp. 140-141). Her understanding of the need for communal support for the individual nurse is reiterated by Muyskens, (1982) who states that it unreasonable to expect individuals to "be heroes" and fight the mores, rules and customs of the system to which they belong. Such behavior taken on without communal support is desirable, a virtue, not a duty.

Professional disobedience is an act taken by an individual nurse, but it is the nursing collective that provides the grounding through community standards and the support through community authority needed by the individual nurse who is professionally disobedient. Collective responsibility can support the individual in situations where the system of health care delivery must be confronted. Because nurses have chosen a profession and have been vested by the states to govern the practice of nursing, nurses as a group have a responsibility to establish within their institutions where they are employed procedures and policies that will support the individual nurse who refuses to participate in practices which lessen the quality of patient care. Nurses, then, no longer have to be heroes when they confront the system, but can be viewed rather as responsible practitioners.

Only through the collective can the profession seek and maintain control of its practice in order to guarantee the quality of its service to the public (Zimmerman, 1978, p. 478). It is only through the collective support of the individual who meets the professional responsibility to the patient through disobedience that nursing can control its practice and assure the quality of the care it provides.

Reconsidering the Professional
Disobedience Guidelines

1. Professional disobedience should only occur when the ethical breach is large. This differs from the duty described in the *ANA Code for Nurses*

(1976) which states that the nurse must safe-guard the patient from *any* unethical or incompetent practice by anyone. Although a principled approach would support the ANA code position, a utilitarian perspective would support limiting professional disobedience to large infractions. "In the interdependent setting that is the modern hospital ... the commitment to work with others is strong. Not just any reason will be sufficient to release one from the obligations to collaborate..." (J. Muyskens, personal communication, February, 1987). Thus, despite the *ANA Code for Nursing* (1976) stance, the interdependency of the hospital practice setting requires that this guideline by Abrams (1980) should remain intact.

2. Normal avenues for correction of the problem should be tried prior to becoming professionally disobedient. In addition, the action should be done openly to shed light on the area of ethical conflict. However, Muyskens pointed out that in certain circumstances, once the normal avenues for correction have been tried and no resolution to the problem has occurred, the nurse is unable to become professionally disobedient. "...To speak openly of (one's) intention *prior* to the act would (be) self-defeating. To confess after the fact hardly would be conducive to change and certainly could put... (the nurse) ...in a weak position to work for that change."

Muyskens relied on a utilitarian justification for not following normal channels openly. In certain cases normal channels do not work. A caring perspective might also support doing what is best for a particular patient, rather than following normal procedures for redress which are likely to be fruitless. However, the principled approach would support the retention of Abrams' (1980) guideline. Although this particular patient may not be helped, the rules which guide practice are confronted, critiqued, and reconfirmed.

The idea of condoning subterfuge and secrecy as methods for achieving ethical results seems almost a contradiction in terms. The concept of accountability, a cornerstone of ethical behavior, is clouded. The balance and validation provided by the nursing community is lost when the nursing action is hidden. The opportunity for individual fallibilism is heightened. When individual nurses act independently to determine both the correct ethical course of action and the feasibility of achieving that course through normal channels, the chances for subjectivism and error increase. The problems that occur with act utilitarianism, especially the lack of trust among co-workers, can result. So, although in a certain situation following normal channels openly may not benefit a particular patient, the guideline for openly following normal channels remains because, overall, it should benefit the greater number of patients.

3. Professional disobedience should not occur if it would break a major ethical principle. Deontological justification for professional disobedience, reveals the fact that Abrams' (1980) third guideline needs modification. Ethical principles such as autonomy and beneficence often do conflict in practice and *any* nursing action, including professional disobedience, may therefore have to break an ethical principle. However, professional disobedience should never occur when it would break the principle of nonmaleficence. When principles support different courses of action, they must be judged and prioritized. The principle of nonmaleficence is the most basic and inviolable. Because the justification for professional disobedience lies in the nurse's primary responsibility to the patient, the nurse cannot justify disobedience when the patient could be harmed.

4. The principles must not just be personal principles, but ones shared by the health care community. This guideline remains but is incorporated into the previous guideline.

The guidelines for professional disobedience have, therefore, been modified as follows:

1. Professional disobedience should occur only when the ethical breach is large.

This guideline remains unchanged.

2. Normal avenues for correction of the problem should be tried and the noncompliance should be done openly. Efforts should be made to make the normal avenues of correction more responsive to the ethical issues.

This guideline is enlarged in scope.

3. Professional disobedience should not occur when a patient's welfare would be jeopardized. It should be justifiable by one of the bioethical principles communally accepted by nurses. One principle may be broken to adhere to another principle when two principles conflict. However, the principle of nonmaleficence cannot be broken.

This guideline is modified and a parameter is set.

Summary

Although reasoning to determine whether an action is ethically justified is necessary for moral discourse, *justification* of actions does not replace the *performance* of the act itself. Simply because professional disobedience is ethically justifiable, does not insure that nurses will be professionally disobedient when the circumstances warrant such behavior. Nursing needs to move beyond justification to judgment and action.

REFERENCES

1. Abrams, N. (1980). "Moral Responsibility in Nursing." In S.F. Spicker & S. Gadow (eds.) *Nursing: Images and Ideals.* (New York: Springer Publishing).
2. American Nurses' Association. (1976) *Code for Nurses with Interpretive Statements.* (Kansas City: American Nurses Association).
3. Aroskar, M. (1982) "Are Nurses' Mind Sets Compatible with Ethical Practice?" *Topics in Clinical Nursing,* 4 (1), 22-32.
4. Aroskar, M. & Veatch, R. (1977) "Ethics Teaching in Nursing Schools." *Hastings Center Report,* 4(4), 23-26.
5. Christy, T. (1973). "New Privileges... New Challenges... New Responsibilities." *Nursing,* 3(11), 3-6.
6. Corwin, R.C. (1961) "The Professional Employee: A Study of Conflict in Nursing Roles." *American Journal of Sociology.* 66, 604-615.
7. Curtin, L.L. (1978) "Nursing Ethics: Theories and Pragmatics." *Nursing Forum,* 17(1), 4-11.
8. Dachelet, C.Z., and Sullivan, J.A. (1979). "Autonomy in Practice." *Nurse Practitioner,* 4, 15-22.
9. Engel, G.V. (1970) "Professional Autonomy and Bureaucratic Organization." *Administrative Science Quarterly,* 12-20.
10. Gilligan, C. (1982). *In a Different Voice.* (Cambridge, MA: Harvard University Press).
11. Gomperz, H. (1939). "Individual, Collective, and Social Responsibility." *Ethics,* 49, 329-342.
12. Jameton, A. (1984). *Nursing Practice: The Ethical Issues* (Englewood Cliffs, NJ: Prentice-Hall).
13. Kalisch, B.J. & Kalisch P.A. (1977). "An Analysis of the Sources of Physician-Nurse Conflict. *Journal of Nursing Administration,* 7, 51-57.
14. Kohnke, M.F. (1982). *Advocacy: Risk and Reality* (St. Louis: C.V. Mosby).
15. Kramer, M. (1982). "Why Does Reality Shock Continue?" In J.C. McClosky & H.K. Grace

(Eds.) *Current Issues in Nursing* (Boston: Blackwell Scientific Publications), 644-653.

17. Labelle, H. (1978). "Nursing Authority." *Journal of Advanced Nursing,* 3, 145-154.

18. Lieberman, B.P. (1973). "The Role of the Nursing Supervisor in Implementing the New Definition of Nursing Practice." *Journal of the New York State Nurses Association,* 4, 39-41.

19. Muyskens, J. (1982). *Moral Problems in Nursing: A Philosophical Investigation* (Totowa, NJ: Rowman & Littlefield).

20. Nuckolls, K.B. (1974). "Who Decides What Nurses Can Do?" *Nursing Outlook,* 22, 626-631.

21. Parsons, M. (1986). "The Profession in a Class by Itself." *Nursing Outlook,* 34, 270-275.

22. Perry, C.M. (1906). "Nursing Ethics and Etiquette." *American Journal of Nursing,* 6, 448-452.

23. Ritter, T., Crulcich, M., and McEntegart, A. (1982) "Nursing Practice: An Amalgam of Dependence, Independence, and Interdependence." In J.C. McClosky and H.K. Grace (Eds.) *Current Issues in Nursing.* Boston: Blackwell Scientific Publications. 5-13.

24. Roberts, J.D. (1986a). "Working with People: Games Nurses Play -- Part I. Merry-go-round and Catch." *American Journal of Nursing,* 86, 848-849.

25. Roberts, J.D. (1986b). "Working with People: Games Nurses Play -- Part II. Pass to a Higher Authority and Trivial Pursuit." *American Journal of Nursing,* 86, 945-946.

26. Stanley, T. (1978). "Nursing." In W. T. Reich (Ed.), *Encyclopedia of Bioethics* (New York: Free Press), pp. 1138-1146.

27. Styles, M.M. (1982). *On Nursing: Toward a New Endowment.* (St. Louis: C.V. Mosby).

28. Walker, D.J. (1983). "Legal Rights and Responsibilities of the Nurse." In N.L. Chaska (Ed.) *The Nursing Profession: A Time to Speak* (New York: McGraw-Hill), pp. 49-59.

29. Walzer, M. (1967) "The Obligation to Disobey." *Ethics,* 77, 163-174.

30. Zimmerman, A. (1978). "Toward a Unified Voice: Individual and Collective Responsibility of Nurses." *Journal of Advanced Nursing,* 3, 475-483.

DISOBEDIENCE IN NURSING
Response to Brody

By James Muyskens
Hunter College - CUNY

Most of the ethical debates in bioethics these days arise from the fact that technology has opened to us options we never had before. We can extend life in ways not possible only a few years ago. The ways we can now modify behavior, transplant organs, enhance functioning, change appearance, produce babies were the stuff of science fiction just a few decades ago. It is not surprising, therefore, that bioethics has focused upon such questions as when we may withhold or withdraw exotic and expensive modes of treatment or how we should pay for and distribute these new, expensive therapies.

As important as these questions are, however, preoccupation with them has caused us to overlook a very different kind of moral quandary faced daily by the hospital staff nurse. Typically the staff nurse must function within an institutional setting that stretches resources to the breaking point. The nurse sees patient care suffer not only because of the shortage of staff and supplies but because of procedural lapses, inadequate guidelines and communication, as well as professional rivalries and personal shortcomings. The new, wondrous technologies may be relevant when considering the plight of the staff nurse; yet if we are to come to terms with the key ethical quandaries facing them, we must turn our attention instead to a rather different question: how can moral obligation be discharged by those "caught in the middle."

As Ms. Brody has pointed out, the staff nurse works in a complex organization in which policy and directives, at least for the most part, are determined by others. Usually the nurse has little or no opportunity to change these policies and directives and as a nurse is not expected to do so and, in fact, is encouraged not to do so. The result is that the conscientious staff nurse suffers professional disillusionment and moral distress.

21

The concept of professional disobedience has been introduced as a means of helping such a nurse. This, of course, is the concept Ms. Brody has analyzed. And her analysis is the subject of this commentary.

What work can the concept of professional disobedience perform? It is introduced to provide a set of criteria for determining both when it is permitted and when it may be obligatory to stand up against those persons or institutional practices that the nurse finds morally offensive. For example, if a physician gives an order that the nurse believes is contrary to the best interests of the patient, under what conditions may he or she or should she or he disobey them?

Ms. Brody is correct in pointing out that our answer to the question will be theory-relative. If our theory of nursing sees the role of the nurse as primarily that of a subordinate, for example, we will adopt a different set of criteria for defensible disobedience than if we see the nurse's role as (say) a patient advocate.

Ms. Brody (following Mila Aroskar) calls the theories of the nurse's role mindsets. She discusses four of them. The first is the traditional role of nurse as subordinate. On this conception, the nurse's role is defined by the duty to act at the behest of the physician. Construed this way, the concept of professional disobedience is inapplicable. "Professional" entails "independent decision making." On this model, the one thing the nurse is not is an independent decision maker.

Interestingly, however, a nurse acting in accordance with this lowly, and perhaps demeaning, conception of the nurse's role may -- in rare instances -- be obliged to disobey a doctor's orders. For example, if a doctor has made an obvious mistake, e.g., she wrote 100 cc's of x rather than the appropriate dosage of 10 cc's, the nurse, as faithful servant, ought not to follow that order. The rationale for disobedience on this model is that following the clearly erroneous order would not serve the doctor well, the one thing the nurse is clearly obliged to do.

22

If, again to draw a contrast, the nurse has a direct responsibility to the patient, as is the case on the patient advocate model, the nurse's obligation not to carry out the physician's order arises from the duty the nurse has to look out for the best interests of the patient. In fact, on the patient advocacy model, the duty to follow physician's orders arises, not from any contractual obligation to the physician, but from the fact that usually carrying out physician directives best serves the patient. In short, the source of the obligation is the nurse's "contractual" obligation to the patient.

Ms. Brody has done an excellent job of presenting the various conceptions of the nurse's role. On the strength of her accounts, we can reject the models that fail to recognize that the nurse's primary duty is to the patient. Surely we can agree as well that the nurse must work cooperatively with the other members of the health care team. Inasmuch as proponents of the patient advocacy model frequently ignore this dimension of modern-day nursing, the advocacy model must be enriched. In short, the nurse, as is also the case with other health professionals, must work for the best interests of the patient. This typically requires both respect for the particular desires and needs of the patient and cooperation with other health professionals to achieve a mutually agreed upon set of goals.

Of course, things don't always work out as intended. Other professionals may not live up to their responsibilities, the procedures adopted may not permit a course of action the nurse considers best for the patient, and so on. Hence, as indicated earlier, the notion of professional disobedience has been introduced to offer guidance when such break-downs occur.

Ms. Brody sets down certain conditions for defensible professional disobedience. These include:

1. The point at issue must be weighty ("the ethical breach" must be "large").
2. Other less drastic measures, including going through normal channels, must have been tried first.

3.	The act of professional disobedience must not result in a breach of other moral duties.
4.	The ethical principle upon which the action is based must be one that is commonly shared by the profession.
5.	The act of professional disobedience must be committed openly.

I propose that we test these conditions by considering an actual case:

> I had worked for several nights in an Intensive Care Unit with a woman who had metastatic cancer. At some point during her illness she refused further chemotherapy and told her family she wanted to stay at home without further treatment until the end came. She went home. However, it became increasingly difficult for her to breathe and one evening a family member took her to the emergency room. She was placed on a respirator without the doctor knowing the basis of the problem. With proper oxygenation, her brain functioned well. But she was furious with everyone. Her arms were restrained and, of course, she couldn't talk, but still she begged with her eyes and hands. I had read her chart, talked with her family, knew the doctor regretted putting her on the respirator but wouldn't take her off. I tried to reason with her and explained her lungs wouldn't function sufficiently without the machine. She understood this but had reached that point when life was unbearable. So, one night when I finished cleaning her, I didn't secure her arm restraints well. She extubated herself and died that night.(1)

Can the actions of this nurse, whom we shall name Ms. Carey, be defended? The patient, Ms. Chance, is being restrained, her hands are tied to protect her from herself and possibly to prevent her from committing suicide. The duty to conserve life appears to require the restraints. Ms. Carey's failure to secure the restraints appears to be a violation of this duty. It also appears to go against a duty many would argue she and other nurses have, namely, a duty to follow the physician's directives, if possible, and, if not, to "remain within channels."

Of course, the putative duty to conserve life and the putative requirement to be a team player are not the whole story. The patient is on the respirator against her wishes. Had her expressed wishes been followed she would either be home or no longer living. She was brought to the emergency room and put on a respirator without her consent; she is being restrained to prevent her from rejecting the unwanted respirator.

Those who support continuing the restraints may suggest that Ms. Chance's resistance is merely a cry for help or no more than a symptom of disorientation, perhaps brought about by oxygen depravation. An account of this sort would provide the rationale for ignoring her pleas and keeping the restraints in place. Ms. Carey challenged the applicability of such an account in this case. She could readily concede that in numerous other cases the account would be appropriate: cases in which patients have not so clearly expressed their desires to forgo hospital treatment and heroics or cases in which patients lack Ms. Chance's awareness and understanding of what is going on. In cases such as the one under discussion, if Ms. Carey is correct, we lack sufficient ground for overriding the strong presumption that patients (as well as other persons) be taken at their word.

Taking Ms. Chance at her word, we can justify the restraints only if we have compelling ground for maintaining that some duty we have, as, for example, our duty to conserve her life, must take priority over respecting her right of self-determination or autonomy. Nurse Carey, in acting as she did, rejected the idea of substituting her judgment or anyone else's for that of Ms. Chance. The consequence was that the duty to respect Ms. Chance's autonomy was given priority even over the duty to conserve her life.

As the various codes of ethics for nurses make evident, a nurse has both the duty to conserve life and the duty to respect the patient's autonomy, uniqueness, and dignity. Where the codes are not clear and where we may find ourselves in disagreement is how we should *order* these duties. That is, we may find it difficult to agree upon which duty should take precedence, when (as in this case) acting in accordance with one duty appears to be incompatible with acting in accordance with the other. Suffice it to say that Ms. Carey came down on the side of patient autonomy over conservation of life. She did this based upon her commitment to patient advocacy as she learned it in nursing school.

Of course, in coming down on the side of autonomy, she went against the judgment of the other health professionals in the case. In doing so, she is taking a step that she must be able to defend. A nurse is only one of several members of a health care team, including other nurses, therapists, and physicians. Patient care in a modern day hospital requires the coordinated efforts of a large number of persons, each assigned, in accordance with training and qualifications, to perform a particular role. In general, if the members of the team providing care do not act in concert (performing their roles in harmony), patient care -- the raison d'etre of the health professions -- will suffer.

In the interdependent setting that is the modern hospital, it is reasonable to expect nurses (as well as other health care professionals) to be team players. This is not a place for the Lone Ranger to thrive. The commitment to work *with* others in order to achieve a common goal must be strong. Not just any reason will be sufficient to release one from the obligations to collaborate that are generated by participation on the team. Reasons such as these are the basis for Ms. Brody's requirement that professional disobedience or going against orders be permitted only in situations in which the evil that would not be redressed without an act of disobedience is grave.

Is this such a case? Can Ms. Carey provide adequate reasons for her decision not to act collaboratively? The case report states that, although the physician regretted having put the patient on the respirator, she would not take her off. Ms. Carey believed she was wrong in this judgment. She gave up on the possibility of changing the doctor's mind and took the matter into her own hands. Clearly in acting as she did, Ms. Carey did not see her role as that of the handmaiden of the physician (a model of the nurse's role that may typify earlier times) or as no more than the physician's surrogate. She acted independently, making her own professional judgment. In fact, she saw herself as having a first or primary allegiance to the patient rather than to the team or the doctor. She was acting, as she herself would say, as a patient or client advocate, and as such she felt obligated to help Ms. Chance exercise her autonomy. As traumatic as it was for her to take an action that could possibly contribute to her patient's death, she believed it was required.

A defense of Ms. Carey's actions requires a demonstration that this duty to support the patient against the coercion of other members of the team outweighs a nurse's duty to collaborate with the team. What would such a defense involve?

We have seen that the putative duty to collaborate arises from general considerations about optimal conditions for patient care. The advocacy requirement is also grounded upon the commitment to patient care. The question we must ask then is whether in this case collaboration or advocacy best meets the basic goal of providing quality patient care. From what has been said, we have a good understanding as to why, when framed this way, Nurse Carey came down on the side of advocacy and why she felt that her duty to act as an advocate for Ms. Chance superceded her duty as a professional to collaborate with the others on the team.

Those who feel the strong pull toward collaboration and the importance of being a team player will feel somewhat uneasy about the form Ms. Carey's advocacy took. Yet they may also recognize that if Ms. Carey had simply gone along with the others, the patient would have been maltreated. What they will look for is a compromise position, one that is less drastic than Ms. Carey's unilateral actions, on the one hand, and, on the other hand, one that is more respectful of the patient as a person than was the doctor's.

They may suggest that Ms. Carey should have refrained from acting upon her own until she had at least another talk with the doctor, hoping to change her mind about the restraints and the respirator. We would need to know more about this doctor to be able to determine whether Ms. Chance gave up on her too quickly. If we are inclined to think she did, we should keep in mind that if further efforts to convince her had failed (and this is certainly a distinct possibility), the one remaining alternative that Ms. Carey had for helping Ms. Chance may have been lost. Similar considerations may have prevented her from taking up the case with her supervisor or with other physicians. Her challenge, she would likely tell us, would have drawn too much attention to her and made the action she later chose either too risky or impossible.

The hospital in which she worked did not have an ombudsman or an ethics committee to whom she could appeal. She could have looked into securing a court ordered "objective" outsider. But she did not. Knowing about the "deliberate speed" of the courts, anticipating that any relief it would grant would be too late, unless the unthinkable happened (Ms. Chance remained in that hospital room tied down and attached to the respirator forty weeks), this option probably did not appear to be a promising avenue for an advocate to take. A creative mind could generate any number of other possible alternatives; but they too -- especially if they remain collaborative -- are likely to do little to offer Ms. Chance relief.

After all is said and done, we are still faced with the question of relative weights of the obligation to work within the system and the obligation to act on behalf of the patient. If a course of action can be found that makes it possible to honor both of these duties, that is the option we should choose. If, by going through channels rather than by taking unilateral action, Ms. Carey could have brought it about that the restraints were removed, she has no defense for having taken matters into her own hands.

28

As we have seen, Ms. Carey (whether rightly or wrongly) saw no way to do that. Being forced to choose, she gave higher priority to advocacy than to collaboration.

Suppose, at least for now, that Ms. Carey was sufficiently diligent in trying to go through channels. Suppose also that she was correct in her judgment that relief for Ms. Chance was possible only if she acted unilaterally. We may still question the way she went about it. We may feel uncomfortable with the fact that she acted secretively. The elements of deception and stealth involved in the case run contrary to the candor and openness we all prefer. If, as Ms. Brody has done, we view Ms. Carey's action as parallel to civil disobedience, we may argue that, if she is going to engage in an act of "professional disobedience," she must do so openly; and she must be willing to accept the consequences of it -- no matter how bad they may be.

Ms. Carey would have to concede that her secretive approach fails to do anything about changing the paternalistic approach to patient care to which she objects. She would also have to concede that it would be wrong to act in this secretive manner if by acting more openly she could have achieved the same end. She can answer the first point by contrasting her basis for action with that of the civil disobedient. The civil disobedient is aiming primarily at changing policy. She is aiming to serve a particular patient. Thus, although a change in policy would be a happy by-product, it is not the aim of her action and so the action ought not to be faulted if it does not result in policy change. With regard to the concern with secrecy, to speak openly of her intention prior to the act would have been self-defeating. To "confess" after the fact would hardly be conducive to change and certainly could put Ms. Carey in a weak position to work for that change.

With our present, perhaps preliminary, convictions about the appropriateness of Ms. Carey's actions as our guide, let's see if the conditions for defensible professional disobedience set out by Ms. Brody seem correct. Her first condition was that the point at issue must be weighty. Our discussion of this case bears this out. The duty to collaborate, we argued, is a strong one not easily overruled. We had more difficulty with her second condition, namely, that the act of disobedience must be one of last resort (i.e., other less drastic measures must have been tried first). Ms Carey chose not to pursue a number of alternatives because she felt that doing so would jeopardize the chances for her unilateral action should they fail. Ms. Brody's third condition (the act of disobedience must not result in a breach of other moral duties) may be too strong. At least as construed by Ms. Carey, she was in a conflict-of-duty situation so that, by engaging in professional disobedience and acting to protect Ms. Chance's autonomy, she couldn't help but violate her *prima facie* duty to conserve life. This third condition just may be too strong to allow any professional disobedience. The fourth condition (that the ethical principle upon which the action is based must be one that is commonly shared by the profession) was satisfied in this case. Ms. Carey was appealing to one of the fundamental principles of the latest ANA code of ethics. Finally, the case under discussion violated the fifth condition (that the action must be done openly). Perhaps a good place to begin our discussion is on this issue: Were you persuaded by the reasoning attributed to Ms. Carey whereby the stealth was defended?

NOTE

1. James L. Muyskens. *Moral Problems in Nursing: A Philosophical Investigation.* (Totowa, New Jersey: Rowman and Littlefield, 1982), p. 135.

ETHICS AND THE HEALTH CARE PROFESSIONAL

By Louis Sportelli, DC

I wish to thank the Long Island Philosophical Society for the kind invitation to participate in this symposium dealing with a most fascinating topic. Ethics is probably the most controversial and confusing subject confronting the health-care practitioner today. My profession, CHIROPRACTIC, has not been spared in the war between ethics and economics, the need to determine where societal responsibility stops and personal interest begins ... or vice versa.

Chiropractic, like all other professions, is struggling with moral values and practical decisions, with "do's" and "don'ts," with "rights" and "wrongs," trying to put hard edges on a subject that is almost jelly-like.

While every profession would like to speak idealistically of being driven by "ethics," all professions find it is a term hard to define and even harder to control. While each of us has a gut feeling about what is ethical and what is not, the dilemma comes in interpretation. The inability to effectively separate the "black hats" from the "white hats" creates frustration which is often vented in anger.

In the past decade, there has been a shift from a controlled health-service environment to a market-driven health-care system. This revolution has produced a fundamental change in the so-called "social contract" between health-care professionals and health-care providers, and between providers and patients. This has put a strain on relationships as effort is made to retain a code of human dedication and social responsibility while maintaining financial stability.

At the same time, new technology and its inherent risks; legal, philosophical and religious aspects; and determinations of personal rights and informed consent, have further distorted the simple moralistic approach to ethics.

Ethics is not easy to define, but let's try. Earl Warren, a former Chief Justice of the Supreme Court, described ethics this way:

"ETHICS IS THE LAW BEYOND THE LAW, WHICH CALLS UPON US TO BE FAIR ... EACH OF US IS NECESSARILY HIS OWN CHIEF JUSTICE: IN FACT, HE IS THE WHOLE SUPREME COURT FROM WHICH THERE IS NO APPEAL."

The word "ethics" is derived from the Greek word *ethos*, which refers to character. Webster defines an ethic as "the discipline dealing with that which is good and bad and with moral duty and obligation."

In general, ethics deals more with good than with evil. A code of ethics tells us what we and others should do. When our ethical codes describe our aspirations rather than our behavior, our ethics are in the process of change. In a sense, whenever ethical practices are codified, they are already in transition, or else putting them into symbolic forms would be unnecessary.

We can also define ethics as a system of moral principles. Our definition could expand to "that branch of philosophy dealing with values relating to human conduct, with respect to rightness or wrongness of certain actions, and to the goodness or badness or the motives and ends of such actions."

It seems the criteria for ethical behavior comes from a number of things. It comes from what we have been taught since our early days about what is right and what is wrong; it comes from an unwritten code established by society; it comes from human instinct; yes, and it comes from religious teachings.

The next logical question then is how do you decide what is RIGHT and what is WRONG? Many people would be satisfied with the concept that ETHICS are a set of MORAL standards that provide guidelines for behavior. Unfortunately, we have come to think of ethics and morals as being synonymous, but they are NOT.

MORALITY simply reflects what the majority is doing. The moralist would argue that if the majority

33

does it, then it is normal. That which is normal reflects what is human, and if what is human is good ... then therefore, we should do what the majority is doing.

That type of thinking is on a direct collision course with everything the BIBLE teaches about GOD, and the undeniable natural laws which govern our universe. Heroes are not taken in by what the majority does, but are committed to what OUGHT to be done, and that is determined not by man, but by a greater power.

MORALITY is doing what we SHOULD do, because it is what our society says it has adopted for itself as the acceptable thing to do.

ETHICS is doing what we OUGHT to do, because it is what God and the fundamental universal laws have set out for us to do.

MORALITY has to do with what we do. ETHICS has to do with what we OUGHT to do. Throughout history heroes are more than moral... they are ETHICAL.

Thus, the question of ETHICS and its role, or should I say changing role, in the health care delivery system will be discussed today. I naturally have a closer relationship with the practice of chiropractic, and thus my comments will be directed toward those practitioners. However, all health-care providers are essentially involved in this deep and often controversial subject, as are other professionals.

Scholars who have studied the subject note that there seems to be a confusion between codes of ethics and codes of professional behavior -- and it applies to all fields: law, business, public relations, accounting, finance, education -- and health-care.

Lucien Matrat states it well when he says, in the *International Public Relations Review*,

> "A code of professional practice governs the behavior of a practitioner in his functional dealings with his colleagues, employees, clients, patients, etc. A code of ethics regulates the behavior which a human being should adopt towards other

human beings. It aims to protect the sacred character of the human person."

He points out that in contrast with a code of professional conduct, which must comply with the laws and customs of each country, codes of ethics are *international* and *universal.* They are timeless. They must be judged in the scope of the sacred character of man, no matter what his race, color, country or faith, and no matter what his or her cultural or social heritage and level.

It has to be recognized that historically, codes of ethics evolved *not* to protect the professions or trade associations that make claim to them as guideposts for their members. Rather, they took their place in human and professional relationships for the sake of the people -- a kind of unwritten rules of conduct.

The key is the establishment of trust and confidence. Man's relations with his surroundings are based on trust. And unless he enjoys the trust, particularly of his advisors, he cannot grow, achieve and enjoy peace of mind and body. Probably this would be the ultimate goal of codes of ethics if they were planned out and written down, which in their original form they were not.

Such is the ultimate goal of a code of ethics in the health-professions -- to respect a certain morality and to win public confidence. Unlike any other code, ethics cannot be established merely by stating it; it must be done by observing it, which involves respecting the principles of both human and social responsibility.

Two of the most discussed ethical questions today regarding the delivery of health-care concern the advertising by health-care providers and the preponderance of practice building/management consultant seminars. Is it ethical to advertise for patients, and if so, how aggressively? Is it ethical to "learn" to gain a greater "profit" out of a practice, to "merchandise" services and to "market" diagnostic and health-care procedures? Recent Supreme Court cases say it is "legal," although it was a no-no for many years. But does being "legal" make it *"ethical"*?

Early in chiropractic's history, the question of advertising by doctors of chiropractic was a major cause of concern. A large segment of the other health-care professionals, who were in the mainstream of the health-care delivery system, formulated opinions regarding the ethics, competence, and professionalism of those practitioners who would elect to advertise. Additionally, other opinion makers of the community, such as community leaders, lawyers, and legislators, considered advertising by doctors of chiropractic to be of questionable value, and certainly professionals who advertised diminished in credibility in the minds of this segment of society.

I don't know if it was right or wrong. I don't even know if it was ethical. But history will show that in the early part of this century, advertising was absolutely necessary for doctors of chiropractic. Who knew chiropractors were effective in treating various health ailments, and more importantly, who was going to tell the public about this new and "unorthodox" profession? Without getting involved in a lengthy discussion about the conspiracy of the American Medical Association to eliminate chiropractic as a health care profession, suffice it to say that the only method left to the solo independent chiropractic practitioner was to employ advertising.

In the *National Journal of Chiropractic*, 1928, author E.M. Taylor, stated

" . . . there will be a chiropractic corpse if we don't amalgamate, organize better, and advertise more. We want the business; let the medical men have the dignity."

The essential message of the time was survival of the profession, at all costs -- dignity or no dignity, ethics or no ethics (which proves that ethics bends when the hunger of survival takes hold). Advertising today, however, is not so much an issue of survival of the profession as it is one which relates to the financial interests of the health-care practitioner. Perhaps one could say the hunger for survival has turned into the pressure of greed.

And so it was, in early chiropractic -- advertising against the then established standard for conduct of so-called "legitimate health-care practitioners" was prevalent. Chiropractic, because of the need to survive, virtually pioneered advertising and public education concepts which were once viewed with disdain. Now, public presentation has become the standard in the health-care industry.

What happened to change the situation was very simple. On June 27, 1977, the U. S. Supreme Court ruled in the *Bates v State Bar of Arizona* that under the limited circumstances, a lawyer has the right under the First Amendment to publish in a newspaper "..truthful advertising concerning the availability and terms of routine legal services." Naturally there was substantial controversy from various members of the Supreme Court, and Justice Burger in particular writing for the minority found it difficult to define "routine" legal services. In 1982 again the Supreme Court ruled that the American Medical Association could no longer prevent its members from advertising.

At first this ruling presented no problems. Most waiting rooms were still full, and most physicians could expect to have a full practice simply by hanging out a shingle. Even though M.D's were allowed to advertise, the practice of actually advertising by a health-care professional carried with it an unethical stigma and unprofessional practice by peers and segments of the public alike.

Editorials appeared in every journal on the pros and cons of advertising. Allan Dyer writing in the *Journal of Medical Ethics*, 1985, 11, pp. 72-78, stated

> "Advertising which provides information to consumers is ethical; creation of the illusion of differences through product differentiation is as unethical in medicine as it is in any other business"

The public, however, can only be expected to assume that information gleaned from an advertisement is truthful and representative of the particular profession for which it is purported to inform. E.

37

Ginzberg stated in the April 8, 1983 *Journal of the American Medical Association:*

> "There is a major asymmetry in the knowledge and judgment of physicians and lay persons, which makes it necessary for the latter to rely on the former for guidance."

The question of advertising then, is relatively a moot one today regarding whether or not a professional should advertise. The only beneficial effect this has had on the chiropractic professional is to remove any stigma from the profession by being singled out as the only advertising professional. For that reason, I am proud to have been in a profession which was in the avant garde of public information by choice, long before the force of the marketplace made advertising mandatory by those professionals who viewed advertising with disdain and now are forced to advertise to maintain their previous level of income.

Over one billion dollars will be spent this year by all forms of health-care providers and various health care facilities on advertising. The question regarding advertising is not whether one should advertise, but in what fashion advertising be done. Will the chiropractic physicians who pioneered the advertising trends for health professionals contain their zeal to escalate the campaign at all costs, or in the words of Irvin Davis, Public Relations Consultant for the American Chiropractic Association:

> "Can chiropractors control themselves while their medical role-models commit image suicide"?

Therein lies the advertising question. How will the advertising by chiropractors today affect the image of the chiropractic practitioners of tomorrow? Will their image be linked to gimmicks such as CROOKED PENS or PICTURES OF GREMLINS BITING SPINES in an attempt to illustrate that spinal ailments are dangerous? Will the advertising continue to depict illustrations of spines and skeletons to

38

illustrate disease, or will the information be that of health and positive public information regarding a holistic approach to health and self-help ideas?

The glut of PHYSICIANS, HMO's, PPO's, DRG's, SELF-INSURED COMPANIES, and GOVERNMENT CONTROLS, all have made the issue of advertising almost as important as clinical skills, as well as a universally accepted practice to attract patients.

The question which must be asked is:

HOW DO WE BALANCE THE DEMANDS FOR FIN-ANCIAL VIABILITY WITH THE TRADITIONAL MISSION OF SOCIAL RESPONSIBILITY?

Or to put it another way:

WILL I, AS A HEALTH CARE PROVIDER, COMPRO-MISE MY OWN PERSONAL STANDARDS OF CONDUCT TO MANAGE A PRACTICE LIKE A BUSINESS?

Not so easy a question to answer by the young doctors graduating with a substantial financial student loan demanding immediate repayment. Couple this with the expense of setting up a practice, the young graduate is vulnerable to many forces, and the lures from those who are offering instant riches and instant practice growth. Thus the second portion of my presentation dealing with practice building seminars and consultants is appropriately staged.

Is there a useful purpose served by practice consultants? Why has the proliferation of practice-building seminars escalated so rapidly in the past few years?

1. There is fierce competition from fellow health care practitioners due to the increase in the number of graduates each year entering practice.
2. There is fierce competition among different providers who essentially treat similar ailments. For example, the physiat-rist/orthopod/chiropractor/physical thera-pist, the obstetrician/midwife/nurse-practitioner, the hospitals and free-standing

surgi-centers -- enough of a blur to make the delineations of services very unclear to the consumer.

3. The education provided in most health care colleges, while good clinically, is totally inadequate to prepare the graduate for the business-like environment of the real world of practice.

Thus the new graduates, and those practitioners who are barely surviving in the cruel world of reality, become easy prey for those unscrupulous entrepreneurs who hold out the promise of riches delivered to your patient in the name of service.

Is this to say that no practice management consultant or seminar is honest or has no value to the practitioner? Of course not. The problem does not come in the vast majority of the necessarily mundane tasks which everyone must do to establish a sound business-like procedure in his/her office, The problem begins when questionable tactics to increase the number of patients, and thus the income of the practitioner, are suggested. The problem comes when clinical procedures are suggested for financial gain rather than clinical necessity. The problem comes when increasing patient visits because of a pre-fixed formula based on the projected income is used rather than on the patient's needs. The problem comes when insurance companies are treated as annuities for the provider rather than benefits and protection for the beneficiary. The problem comes when diagnostic equipment is purchased because it has an ICDA or CPT number for billing purposes vs. a justifiable reason for purchase based upon patient benefits.

There must be a blend of ethical considerations and managerial decisions if the consumer is truly to be protected from a practitioner who is entrusted with the health decisions. The demand for health care is insatiable, and unlike oil or copper or gold which essentially have limited utility, health is life, and how can you have too much of either?

Allen Dyer commenting in the *Journal of Medical Ethics*, 1985, (11) pp. 72-78 stated

"To the extent that medicine relies merely on technique and not on an ethic of service, it becomes merely a trade and not a profession."

The same can be said of chiropractic if we as a profession lose sight of our true purpose -- to treat the patient and not just the disorder. We could, under those limitations, lose the right to call ourselves professionals.

Is the profession of chiropractic a business? Certainly, and as noted by E. Pellegrino in the 1984 *Survey of Ophthalmology,*

"Healing is something more than a commodity transfer. ... All the healing professions demand not the ethos of the marketplace, but rather ... the ethics of virtue."

By far the vast majority of chiropractic physicians can recognize and have a code of professional ethics. Ethics, however, cannot be regulated by law, but must be self-regulated. To date, however, self-regulation has had little effect on controlling the flamboyant, questionable advertising practices of many health providers, nor has self-regulation satiated the appetite to attend practice building seminars. As long as health care professionals are lured towards questionable seminars, the problem will continue to exist.

Some might ask about now, "What would be considered questionable practices which are taught at some seminars?" I'll give you a few examples of conduct unbefitting an ethical health-practitioner, be he a chiropractor or a medical doctor. But unfortunately, there are some (although a very small percentage) who use these unsavory tactics.

1. Circling the doctor's name with a grease pencil in all telephone books found at public pay phones.
2. Having the receptionist make "phantom" calls asking if they have the office of Dr. so and so,

41

and then proceeding to tell the other person about the wonderful qualifications of the doctor.

3. Marking on the back of a business card, as if the patient is writing a note to a friend, indicating how much the doctor has helped his/her headaches, backaches, etc.

4. Never telling patients they are cured because they may not continue to come back.

5. Having double standards of charges -- one for the insurance company and one for paying patients.

6. Publishing no "out-of-pocket expense," and then padding the bill to recoup the loss.

7. Advertising "free" services as a bait and switch come on, only to charge the patient for other items.

8. Having a re-examination procedure set up in advance for insurance purposes and adhering to it regardless of clinical justification.

The list could go on, but the important point to recognize in the discussion of practice-building seminars, is that they have now become almost an integral part of the health-care professional's education. As a result, the individual practitioner tends to view involvement in practice-building activities with the same seriousness as applied to the study of anatomy and physiology.

The doctor must raise a level of ethical conscientiousness which is to be used as the benchmark for those procedures he/she will employ in practice.

In dealing with ethics, we find ourselves also dealing with value systems -- the values of the professional practitioner himself and the values of the patients or clients. The professional cannot afford to leave his or her value system at home when opening the door of his office. The same values that apply to his family and loved ones must also apply to his patients. As a health-care practitioner, it is my duty to respect my patients' anatomy, mind, soul and reputation. As Reverend Kevin D. O'Rourke of St. Louis University Medical Center states:

"The relationship between patients and health-care professionals penetrates to the very heart of what makes us human: our conscience. Building relationships with each person, both patient and professional, is a task that bespeaks the transcendent worth of health care."

The deeper you study ethics, the more you note that ethical concepts do not fit into neat textbook situations. It is not a matter of choosing the obvious good over the obvious bad. Anyone can do that. The trouble is that the alternatives are often almost equally worthy.

Some practices, like lying, cheating, and stealing, might give us initial advantages. Yet, we realize that if everybody behaved that way we would develop into a society of hermits. Therefore, the ethical precepts: No lying, no cheating, no stealing.

But, what about the white lie for the sake of the hospital patient dying of cancer, or for his wife? What about the person who steals a loaf of bread to keep his family or himself alive? The speaker who plants questions in the audience? Or the doctor who takes a course in "the profitability of diagnostic testing"?

According to the American Society of Association Executives Handbook, four main ethical theories that overlap explain how man has developed his ideas of what is good or bad. The person who seeks to systematize his ethics should be familiar with these major approaches.

Empirical theory takes the stand that ethics is derived from human experience and is conceived by general agreement, like banning certain weapons of warfare.

Rational theory says that through reason we determine what is good or bad. These logical determinations are more or less independent of experience since the values exist in perfect form. Reason simply enables us to approximate the perfect. Plato, Aristotle, and Spinoza were proponents of this theory.

Intuitive theory suggests that ethics are not necessarily derived from experience or logic. Rather, humans automatically or instinctively possess an understanding of right and wrong. This is the doctrine of "natural moral law."

Revelation theory places the determination of right and wrong above man. It holds that God tells man about the principles by which life can attain its greatest potential. The first 200 years of American history are intertwined with the revelation theory of ethics. As the Word of God, the Bible was infallible in matters of conduct. Another segment of revelation theory holds that God continues to make ethical decisions.

Whether we adhere to an empirical theory, a rational theory, an intuitive theory, a revelation theory, or all four, we know that the oldest traditional value in health care is *compassion*. This is born out of an understanding that there is terror in pain and the unknown of disease ... and taking that further, death. That was true a thousand years ago, and it will be true a thousand years from now. Thus, the chiropractic physician of today and tomorrow, or any practitioner for that matter, regardless of the definition placed upon him/her, regardless of the education mandated in his/her studies, must always insure that he/she practices with integrity in the mind, and compassion in the soul.

The present high-tech environment has stimulated many new efficiencies and innovations. It has proven that we as health-care providers can adapt to change and still deliver quality care if we want to. Further change lies ahead.

But while innovation is fundamental to progress, this does not mean a value-free society is permissible. The rights and dignity of man is a spirit that must permeate the professions. They must guide our consciences and our movements as we administer to our patients and our clients. We must recognize that "ethics" is that fragile fiber that separates man from beast, and professional from exploiter.

Mindful of man's dignity, it is that spiritual and moral spark that ties training and experience into a wrap of conscientious public service. Ethics is the wisdom of the ages, the courage of our convictions, the temperance of what is good for us, the justice of human rights, the conscience of sensitivity ... the VOICE OF GOD.

THE SOCIAL CHARACTER OF MEDICAL ETHICS
Reply to Sportelli

By Richard E. Hart[1]
Bloomfield College

Dr. Sportelli's stimulating essay has obviously evolved from prolonged and intense self-reflective medical practice. It offers a healthy and useful mixture of ideals and practicalities, the purely theoretical and the unabashedly concrete. It deals in confusion and controversy and invites serious discussion of central ethical concerns that arise in everyday medical practice. In this spirit I wish to take up its challenge and expound upon areas where I agree and disagree.

In four basic areas I generally agree with Sportelli, though I think it useful to expand or modify his analysis somewhat. 1) The key to the conduct of a medical professional, according to Sportelli, "is the establishment of trust and confidence" with the client/patient. Moreover, codes of ethics in the health professions should serve primarily as a catalyst to the realization of this trust and confidence. Too often these essential traits characterizing the basic relationship between caregiver and client are conveniently overlooked in discussions of medical ethics. Furthermore, they may become all but lost in the exigencies of the day to day business of health care delivery. Sportelli questions, for example, whether there can be compatibility between the achievement of basic client trust and confidence and the commonplace practices of medical advertising and practice building seminars. Do such activities reinforce, enhance or detract from the realization of these desired relationships? From the vantage point of ethics, there's no question that Sportelli is asking the right questions.

---

[1]Reprinted with permission of the American Chiropractic Association; *ACA Journal*, May 1987 issue, Vol. 24, No. 5.

2) For Sportelli, ethics ultimately boils down to self-regulation and personal values, or as he occasionally says, conscience and individual character. This understanding is, of course, part of a long standing tradition. Therefore, ethics, in a medical setting, is absolutely contrary to mere technique ("to treat the patient and not just the disorder"). One's ethics, he claims, cannot be regulated by law or other forms of externally imposed regulation. One's personal values (in relation to family and loved ones) must be synonymous with the values enacted in the medical context. Sportelli bolsters this position by citing former Supreme Court Justice Earl Warren who offered the metaphor of each of us serving as our own Chief Justice. While Sportelli is not incorrect in focusing his inquiry at the level of the individual practitioner, in today's environment this is inevitably only part of the story. In my view, ethics in the realm of health care is wholly inseparable from its societal implications, from public policy and funding issues, legislation and the activities of courts and professional medical societies. I shall focus directly on these themes later in my response.

3) Sportelli is admirably sensitive to the formidable, practical challenges to ethics presented in daily health care delivery. He highlights the delicacy of this matter when, for example, he contrasts economics and ethics. Indeed, his statements perhaps unwittingly reveal more of the danger and ambivalence in this realm than he realizes. For example, he discusses historically the conspiracy of the A.M.A. against the existence of chiropractic medicine and proudly defends the long-standing practice of advertising as necessary to the very economic survival of chiropractic as a profession. In citing a 1928 article in *The National Journal of Chiropractic*, Sportelli quotes E.M. Taylor as saying, "We want the business; let the medical men have the dignity." But, as Sportelli knows, this is precisely the rub. Chiropractic doctors, as well as others, hopefully want the business and the dignity. Can we have both economic survival and ethical conduct? In today's competitive marketplace for health care services, can these two goals co-exist or does one tend to in-

evitably undermine the other, creating either the impoverished, ethical doctor or the immoral, perhaps amoral but wealthy, huckster? Is there a weakness in man, the system, the laws or codes, the training? Sportelli suggests, but does not intensely confront or resolve, the ambivalence and uncertainty surrounding these questions today. For instance, he describes the precarious financial circumstances confronted by young doctors, indeed, all caregivers, today and concludes that advertising and consultant seminars have probably become an imperative for survival. At the same time, he realizes, from an ethical standpoint, that "the hunger for survival has turned into the pressure of greed." So where is the line drawn? Can a balance be struck between the necessity of financial viability and the imperative to act ethically? On principle, it should be possible. In practice, it seems unusually difficult, which helps to explain, though not justify, why an alarming number of health care providers have obviously either missed the mark or given up the quest entirely. It's comforting to think that individual professional ethics will ride in on a white horse and save the day, but is this an exercise in wishful thinking? As Sportelli muses, "...ethics bends when the hunger of survival takes hold." I question what role must be played by the courts, the lobbyists, media campaigns publicizing wrongdoing, public education programs, or, in short, critical public debate. While individual conscience should be the ultimate regulator of such matters, conscience may well be in a state of collective debilitation in today's often amoral world.

4) From among many possible options, Sportelli identifies what he terms two highly significant ethical issues faced by today's practitioner, namely, advertising and use of practice building seminars and consultants. Sportelli is correct I believe in characterizing the shift in recent years "from a controlled health-service environment to a market-driven health-care system." This tends to bring about a critical change in the "social contract" between providers and clients, calling into question the dedication and responsibility of the individual health care professional. As Sportelli aptly points out, Supreme

Court rulings have made advertising of health care services legal, but it may still, in some cases, be unethical. The legal vs. ethical distinction is crucial here. While advertising seems to be evolving as a necessary feature of a successful practice, the essential question concerns the truthfulness of the advertising. Consumer fraud is a violation of law, whereas basic deception of the lay public is a breach of trust and confidence, a violation of ethics.

Similar arguments could be waged as regards the preponderance of practice building consultants and seminars. Sportelli cites an alarming number and variety of practices that can become the bi-products of actualizing consultant's recommendations: questionable practices to increase the number of patients, unnecessary clinical procedures, pre-fixed formulas of projected income needs vs. patient needs, double standards of charges, etc. As competition becomes more intense, and economic viability less certain, the "blend of ethical considerations and managerial decisions" may become skewed, unbalanced, and seemingly unachievable.

Again Sportelli analyzes these issues primarily in terms of the individual provider's ethical obligations and the potential erosion of the glue that makes the health care system work, that is, trust and confidence. I hasten to mention, however, at least one of the long-range societal implications that extends beyond the breakdown of provider-client trust. Sportelli claims that one billion dollars will be expended this year in advertising for health care services and facilities. Additionally, consultants and seminars are obviously becoming a more prominent expense item for providers. The costs of these activities inevitably are passed along to consumers in the form of higher fees for services. A ripple effect takes hold with all the attendant consequences for insurance companies, government programs, employer-sponsored benefit packages, etc. This simply confirms once again how ethical issues in health care practice inevitably extend beyond relationships between individual persons, reaching out to assimilate a myriad of factors and activities that orbit around these fundamental relationships. In my view, this is one of the reasons why the bio-medical and health service areas represent the most enduring and controversial public debates in our society, both today and in the foreseeable future.

As regards disagreements with Sportelli, some rather strong hints have already been proffered. Basically, I find myself questioning two aspects of the paper. I shall elaborate on each briefly.

Sportelli and I have different conceptions of what I will term the "nature of ethics". He alludes to ethical behavior stemming from such sources as parental teachings, societal codes and human instinct. But the higher view of ethics, which he ultimately seeks to defend, incorporates God, religious teachings and what he calls "universal natural laws". In his final sentence he refers to ethics as, among other things, "the VOICE OF GOD." Based on his categorical delineation of types of ethical theories (empirical, rational, intuitive, and revelation) the reader must conclude that the revelation theory is the most compelling for Sportelli. Ethics, thus, becomes the great divider, that which separates man from beast, exploiter from professional, man from God.

As we all know, ethicists have long challenged the defensibility of the revelation and/or natural law theories of ethics, inasmuch as they are claimed by their advocates to be exclusively binding on human conduct. While questions of confirmation, verifiability, faith vs reason abound, I don't wish to take up space here rehashing time-honored debates. I do wish, however, to briefly contrast my approach to the nature of ethics with that of Sportelli's in hopes that further thought and discussion might be thereby facilitated. My understanding of ethics I will call "contextualist". It grows out of the Pragmatist tradition in American philosophy and is probably championed most prominently in the works of John Dewey. Using Sportelli's categories, the "contextualist" approach unites rational theory and empirical theory in a novel and productive synthesis. It is rooted in the challenges of man's unique and ever-changing experience, and takes as fodder for reflection all the relevant traits and possibilities that characterize any context in which we find ourselves.

Reasoning (of the valuing sort) is applied to any specific context in an open-ended, unprejudiced manner. Any ethical context reflects a dilemma, an ethical dilemma. Reason seeks its terminus in decision and subsequent action. Ethical principles, societal codes, religious teachings, parental influence, all can function as aids to the process of reasoning though none necessarily represent answers within themselves. While they help orient and guide the deliberation, they rarely function as stop-signs. As Professor Evelyn Shirk, a defender of contextualism in ethics, has asserted, "Ethical choice becomes meaningful only when seen as the choice of some valuer who selects one option as against other possible options within a particular context". Furthermore, under this view "...we have lost absolute values and immutable standards for the measurement of good." (1)

When considering Sportelli's examples of advertising and practice building consultants, he and I might well reach similar conclusions regarding the ethicality of such practices, but undergo very different reasoning in the achievement of our conclusions. Our ends could be common but our means different. In other contexts, we might well agree or disagree on both counts. Whereas Sportelli might disagree ethically with excesses in these practices on grounds that they violate God-ordained trust, I might well argue that, in this or that specific situation, the overriding factor is that costs to consumers become burdensome and unfair, or people are being treated as means rather than ends, or dangerous public policy precedents are being established. The focus of my assessment of the situation is flexible though not unprincipled, chaotic or irrational. Rather it is critical and realistic, emerging out of man's desire to resolve the dilemmas he finds himself in.

A "contextualist" understanding of ethics has further implications that I alluded to earlier and which will be my second point of disagreement. For Sportelli, medical ethics is primarily rooted in personal values, the decisions and actions of the individual. While I can't wholly disagree, I fear that this view is ultimately too narrow and impractical. It places too heavy a burden squarely on the shoulders of the individual and that person's wherewithal, sense of professionalism and responsibility. Without underestimating the importance of responsible individual conduct, a "contextualist" accepts and looks for all the influences and ramifications built into situations that impact on people. When considering any serious issue of medical ethics, on one level the relevant decisions and conduct are very much individual. On another equally important level, we cannot overlook the role of legislation, public policy, funding, and other political and economic variables. Virtually any case involving medical ethics, whether abortion, euthanasia, surrogate motherhood or advertising, affects the interests of the public at large. Individual actions are rarely sufficient in tackling the problems. Courts must adjudicate disputes, legislation must be considered to curtail certain practices, governments must decide to cut-off or enhance funding for various programs. These are the practical realities of our complex, interrelated world. This reflects the interface, the confrontation, between the practical and the ethical, a matter which even Socrates, in his time, knew something about.

In the end, I favor pulling out all the stops in the effort to achieve a fair and open assessment of today's medical practices, and in the hopes that we, as individuals and as a society, end up doing what is morally right. For example, I favor required ethics courses in all types of medical and nursing training programs. Controversial though it may seem, I favor an ethics component on licensing exams for medical professionals. I advocate open, and heated, public debate on issues of medical ethics and extensive media condemnation of wrongful practices and the rogues who perpetrate them. I support lawsuits and court hearings and, if necessary, legislation that rules out or severely limits certain practices, like that now being considered in relation to surrogate parenting. I believe professional societies should develop clear, coherent codes of conduct and strive to see that their members comply. While my list of suggestions could go on, I hope my multi-barreled attack on the problems of medical ethics has become clear. In short, we have to work on the individual, on our laws, our institutions all at once. Anything less spells potential failure.

All of this is prerequisite I believe to achieving the balance that Sportelli cites as the goal and which I heartily agree with, that is "...the blend of ethical considerations and managerial decisions" or financial viability and traditional social responsibility. As he wisely points out, in today's environment the question is not whether there should be advertising or consultant seminars. The question is, What kinds of advertising? To what extent? What sorts of managerial practices? We can come closer to having our cake and eating it too, but if, and only if, we keep the theme of balance in focus as individuals and as a society. For Sportelli, this balance is ultimately to be achieved through the individual's recognition of universal natural laws and God. For me, it's more a matter of a secularized business proposition. We need negotiated settlements, one eye forever focused on the morally good, the other on the mundane practical facts and challenges of this world. In other words, what we ought to do is finally determined by man. On my view, the Dr. Sportellis of the world represent the thesis, the consultant/hucksters and Wall Street "inside traders" the anti-thesis. Probably somewhere in between lies the achievable synthesis, the best we can get.

NOTE

1. Shirk, Evelyn.   *The   Ethical   Dimension* (Appleton Century Crofts, 1965), p. 13.

THE WELLNESS MOVEMENT AND VICTIM BLAMING

By Beth Furlong, R.N., M.S.
Creighton University

The wellness movement, a preventive health phenomenon of both the health care system and of the larger United States' society, is of recent origin (Laughlin, 1982; Fielding and Breslow, 1983). While it has many positive aspects, including better individual health status indicators and is one method of containing health care costs, there are also some negative aspects to this movement. This paper will address the shadow side of the wellness movement with particular focus on the concern of victim blaming being associated with it. This author agrees with Allegrante and Green (1981) who raised a concern that an ideology of individual responsibility could preach an elite moralism while failing to recognize or ignoring the political, economic, or environmental forces that mold and reinforce behavior. At the worst it could divert attention and responsibility away from addressing such social forces. They note that without organizational, economic, and environmental supports for wellness behavior, promoting health education for individual responsibility can be a smoke screen for cost containment.

The wellness movement is characterized by being of recent origin -- the past five to ten years have been noteworthy by both the increased consciousness of individuals and the increased number of programs available to individuals and in the worksite (Fielding and Breslow, 1983). A review of the literature with the vast number of articles and books on this topic is another indicator. Although preventive health issues have always been with us, the recent particular focus is different and of greater importance.

The following reasons have been given for the emphasis on the wellness movement now: 1) A major reason is the escalating cost of health care in our society. The wellness movement, with its emphasis on preventive health, is viewed as one important strategy to prevent illness and therefore to decrease the overall cost of the health system (O'Donnell and Ainsworth, 1984). It is recognized that it may or may not have immediate cost reduction but it is an important long term strategy. This is because of the longer timeline for causation and appearance of symptoms of chronic illnesses. 2) There has been a significant change in the causes of morbidity and mortality in the United States in the past seventy-five years (Stanhope and Lancaster, 1984). In essence, there has been a dramatic shift from illness and death caused by communicable and infectious diseases to those caused by what is termed "lifestyle" diseases and/or chronic diseases. In public health, the paradigm for viewing disease is the triad of environment, agent, and host (Wilner, *et al.*, 1973). During the Era of Bacteriology, the emphasis was on the agent, i.e., the causative organism. During certain historical periods, the emphasis was on the environment, i.e., at the turn of the century, there was emphasis placed on environmental sanitation and safe water, milk, and food supplies (Archer and Fleshman, 1985). During the 1970's there was emphasis on passage of federal laws that decreased environmental pollution (Archer and Fleshman, 1985). The wellness movement is one indication that in the 1980's, the emphasis is on the host, i.e., man. Some wellness advocates paraphrase Pogo, "We have met the enemy, and he is us," because they see the linkage between the chronic illnesses and lifestyle causation. Thus, they problem solve by focusing on one part of the triad -- man, the host. 3) Another major reason for the interest in prevention is the surge in research studies and knowledge in this area. Einstein's discovery of relativity is seen as a historical water-shed in terms of its impact on the integration of research that pertains to mind, body, and spirit (Flynn, 1980). In addition, the past forty years have been marked by prolific research and an increased understanding of holistic man (Blattner, 1981). 4) A final reason given for the present interest in wellness is the "California effect." Two aspects of wellness-- physical fitness and holistic healing methodologies-- are correlated with having started in California, and then influencing the rest of the country.

Numerous articles and books have been written which speak to the benefits of the wellness movement (Flynn, 1980; Blattner, 1981; O'Donnell and Ainsworth, 1984). Five major benefits will be addressed here: 1) it may decrease morbidity and mortality; 2) because of the first benefit, it may reduce total costs spent on health care; 3) better health status indicators for the individual; 4) in the work setting, there may be increased productivity, decreased absenteeism, etc.; and 5) for the individual there may be more opportunity for the attainment of his potential, i.e., one may be more able to achieve one's maximum growth. This results not only in positive outcomes for an individual and his family, community, and country-- but, also, in a larger global sense, for all of humanity.

But concomitant with the benefits are three ethical issues: 1) paternalism versus autonomy; 2) distributive justice; and 3) victim blaming. The remainder of this paper will address in detail concerns with the latter. However, limited attention will be paid to the second one, especially because it also relates to the latter concern.

There are many concepts applicable to the wellness movement and a plethora of specific wellness behaviors. However, the one core concept that has ramifications for the concern for victim blaming is this one -- the individual is responsible for his health status. Ardell, considered one of the first advocates of wellness, writes, "All dimensions of high level wellness are equally important, but self-responsibility seems more equal than all the rest... Self-responsibility represents your keystone to a life of high level wellness (1977). It is such a concept -- if held dogmatically -- that can lead to victim blaming.

Victim blaming refers to attitudes held or behaviors demonstrated by health providers toward patients, individuals with each other, and citizens and administrators, et al., who make health policy in the public and private sectors, that results in attitudes and actions where an individual is blamed for causing his illness.

A blaming-the-victim mentality is not restricted to the health system. It is a way of problem identification and problem solving in other aspects of our society too. For example, it is only in the past five to ten years that the paradigms of thinking have changed for the causation of rape and abuse (Campbell and Humphreys, 1984). Prior to this shift in paradigm thinking and research, such individuals were blamed for inviting the rape or abuse. Other authors would point to societal attitudes that blame the poor for their place in society. Although not victim blaming *per se*, research done by Bordieri, *et al.* (1985) reports on a related facet. The study investigated the effect of physical attractiveness of pediatric patients on nurses' impressions. Less attractive patients were viewed in a more negative manner. This author believes that there could be an analogy to individuals who don't meet all the external criteria of visible wellness behaviors. Vanderhaar writes about scapegoating, which is analogous to victim blaming: "Scapegoating is not the best way to face life. But it's a pattern most people fall into fairly frequently, because it's a remarkably effective short term remedy for anxiety" (Vanderhaar, 1985, p. 7). Victim blaming with the wellness movement could be a short term remedy for anxious concerns about escalating health care costs.

It is a concern of this author that such victim blaming may be a negative spin-off of the wellness movement. The cost containment ideology of the 1980's could serve as an impetus to such a way of viewing patients. Thus, we're at an unique convergence timewise -- the wellness movement and cost-containment. Blaming the victim may be a strategy when frustrated with declining resources for health care. This author agrees with Pellegrino in viewing a patient as "wounded humanity" and views a blaming-the-victim mentality as antithetical to the healing relationship between provider and patient (1983). However, the implications go beyond the healing relationship between health provider and patient. There are definite ramifications for the societal milieu -- how patients with certain diseases are viewed, and what kind of health policy decisions are made by those having the power to do so in both the public and private sectors. The private sector is highlighted here because of its increasing importance -- especially relative to wellness at the worksite. Iglehart has also noted, "Private businesses, foundations, and universities are not alone, though, in shifting their attention to communities and away from Washington's policy swirl in pursuit of reforming health care delivery. So, too, are a tiny cadre of persons who once viewed Washington as the place where medical care could be transformed through broad strokes of national policy" (Iglehart, 1982, p. 123). Thus, policy refers to both public and private sectors.

Many examples of a shift to victim blaming exist. Several will be cited. First, Connelly writes "although less common than occasional or episodic noncompliance, persistent noncompliance poses an ethical dilemma to nurses that directly raises questions about the economic implications of this behavior. Is the provision of care to individuals who seem intent on ignoring repeated discussions and warnings about the consequences of noncompliance ethically and economically justified?" (1984, 344). It should be noted that this article did not greatly emphasize whether the nurse had exhausted all motivational strategies, methods, etc. to help the patient. Rather, the above quote seems to succinctly capture the cost containment philosophy of the mid-1980's. A second example is taken from a local vendor of fitness programs. The following statements are taken from printed materials describing services that his organization can offer. Along with employment screening, he offers a "Pre-Employment Back Examination." "The Pre-Employment Back Examination is intended to discover those individuals who have a predisposition to developing back problems *before they're on your payroll* (his italics). The exam includes the following...". Further content states that the role of this vendor is to "Provide employers with the above information and make recommendations." The unstated but implicit implication for the above is that the individual will be held responsible for his back problem and probably not be hired. From a financial point of view one can appreciate this from the employer's perspective since a major expense in Workman's Compensation is for back injuries (Lee *et al.*, 1983). However, this is one example when blaming the victim can result in job discrimination.

Third, at a wellness seminar, a national leader in health promotion spoke to the choices that companies had to make in budgeting resources for company wellness programs. He spoke that it could be a "Cadillac" operation and be inclusive of all employees or that many companies would have to make the decision to have such programs available only to upper management. The concern of this author is that later company policies would be promulgated that would result in victim blaming for the employees who didn't change their behaviors (but also didn't have access to such helpful programs). It again raises the issue of distributive justice. It also raises the issue that in some settings the wellness programs are not being targeted at those most in need. A fourth example is not hiring smokers for selected jobs. Of irony to this author is the incongruence being demonstrated, especially in the work setting, of an attitude toward the alcoholic and the smoker. Both are addictive diseases (Palin and Ravenholt, 1984). However, business and industry has a positive history of use of employer assistance programs for treatment and rehabilitation of alcoholics. The philosophy is to help rather than dismiss them. This author's analysis is that we're not at that stage yet with the smoker. Rather, the smoker is perceived as lacking will power and can thus be blamed. Alcoholics used to be viewed in the same manner until health providers and the lay public recognized that alcoholism was a disease. Smoking is also an addictive disease. Because of the strength and the rapid growth of the wellness movement, this author questions if all health providers and the public will be educated soon enough on the addictive quality -- rather, in this instance, victim blaming may occur first. Many more examples could be cited. However, most are occurring, and this author believes, will continue to occur in these areas -- job discrimination, access to health systems, financial penalties relative to payment of health care, private and public sector health policies, and in attitudes toward them by health providers and other individuals.

Five reasons why it is incorrect and dangerous to put all the emphasis on self-responsibility will be listed and discussed.

First, disease is multi-causational (Stanhope and Lancaster, 1984). Multi-causational factors could include any of the following -- genetic, congenital, infectious, radiation, habits, environmental pollutants, occupational hazards, the interplay and synergism of several factors, the individual uniqueness of the individual with all that entails, etc. It is obvious that an individual can't control all these variables. Thus, the core concept becomes muddied.

Second, Navarro's research analyzes the correlation of social class standing with individual health status indicators (Navarro, 1976). He posits that one can't study a health system without studying the larger economic system from which it emanates. His research exemplifies well the inverse correlation between morbidity and mortality and social class standing from an epidemiological perspective. Social class standing determines/influences what profession/job one enters and thus the occupational hazards to which one is exposed. There is a direct relationship between occupational hazards and jobs held by individuals in the lower socio-economic classes. Thus, simply because of the way a social class structure works, the health status of individuals is affected. Hence, the multi-causational aspect is again underscored.

Third, if one subscribes to the mental health concept (which this author does) that all behavior has meaning, then one views an individual from a different stance than that of victim blaming (Wilson and Kniesel, 1979). One accepts the individual, in a Judeo-Christian or humanistic system, and doesn't condone the illness behaviors, but recognizes, for this moment in time, that this illness behavior has meaning and is meeting a need. This philosophy doesn't endorse rationalization or denial of their behavior, does allow for working toward changing the illness to a wellness behavior, and, most importantly, promotes acceptance of the individual versus nonacceptance and victim blaming.

Fourth, the work by Milio (1981) recognizes the importance of macro structures as both a causation of illness behavior and a method of problem solving for wellness behaviors. She analyzes that individuals are efficient with their time, money, and energy in relation to the benefits they will gain. Individuals may choose or habitually practice illness behaviors because it is most efficient for them with their time, money, or energy given their perception of benefits. If one agrees with this analysis, it gives emphasis to the third reason -- that all behavior has meaning-- and leads one to a non-victim blaming stance.

A fifth reason why victim blaming is not indicated is the body of research done on the reasons for noncompliance with health behaviors (Geller, 1981; Pender, 1975; Hallal, 1982; Gochman, 1974; Dracup, 1982; Laufman, 1978; Hochbaum, 1982; Steckel, 1977; Lowery, 1976). Studies in the early 1970's demonstrated alarming rates of noncompliance (Connelly, 1984). In a review of research studies, approximately thirty-three patients were noncompliant. Major reasons given for noncompliance were: 1) poor comprehension; 2) social and environmental factors; 3) characteristics of the regimen; and 4) characteristics of the relationship between the provider and the patient. The following two statements are significant for a health provider's attitudes and actions. "Inattention to an individual's life situation and failure to tailor regimens to their needs and resources do not meet professional standards of practice. The quality of the relationship between the patient and the health care provider has been demonstrated to have a significant impact on continued compliance" (Connelly, 1984, 344) What happens many times-- which is demonstrated empirically and reflected in the literature -- is that some health care providers become frustrated, ignore the above, and slip into the ideology of blaming the patient (Murphy, 1982). In essence, it may be easier for the health care provider; he doesn't have to expend as much energy. Milio has also written on the difficulty of changing people's behaviors -- especially since the wellness movement focuses on difficult to change areas-- smoking, obesity, drinking, etc. One of her arguments has special cogency -- we all do the best we can at any one time. Thus, her philosophy correlates with the mental health concept -- that all behavior has meaning. She recognizes and affirms that individuals be helped toward change -- but that it be done in a positive tolerant way. One of the ironies about victim blaming is that if one subscribes to a wellness model that integrates mind, body and spirit, then such judgementalness is an illness and not a wellness behavior. One example will exemplify this -- at a Nebraska state health department meeting on health promotion, an expert physical fitness leader aggressively and dogmatically advocated that all pregnant women who were ingesting alcohol at cocktail parties be arrested.

The above five reasons are important considerations to keep in mind when reflecting on the wellness movement and possible victim blaming. However, there are also other factors that need to be addressed, especially as they correlate with the first, second, and fourth reasons -- multi-causality of disease, correlation of social class with incidence of disease, and the impact of macro structures on illness.

A recent study (Taylor and Thoma, 1985) points to the interplay of modernization of a country's economy and how a changing way of life can be correlated with an increase in the lifestyle-induced chronic illnesses. Their study of Nauru, a small island in the Central Pacific, has different morbidity and mortality statistics compared to other similar populations. Their interpretation is that the statistics are correlated with socio-economic development variables. Are individuals to be blamed for their illnesses because they live in a historical time when their country is in transit from one stage of development to another?

There are many illnesses caused by environmental hazards that need to be addressed. Does one blame the individual living in Missouri at the time of the dioxin spill who later develops cancer? Or the Nevada resident who was exposed to radiation during the 1950's? Or should they have been bolstering their immune systems throughout this time period by visual imagery? Iglehart analyzes well the many faceted problems of smoking and public policy (Iglehart, 1984).

Such questions as these raise two interlocking concerns. The first is the changing body of knowledge and the second is the changing rules of society. There are numerous and increasing epidemiological studies that correlate certain diseases with risk factors, etc. However, a negative aspect of this almost overwhelming plethora of research is the facet of contradictory research findings. This can have direct implications in victim blaming. For example, one may behave or change behavior to correlate with research findings so that one can practice as many wellness behaviors as possible. However, during one's later life, new research may prove the earlier theory incorrect.

Students of the history of public health and medicine will recognize the changing treatment and self care modalities. And although one smiles with amusement at thought patterns in 1785 or 1885, one can predict that the sophistication thought to be true in 1985 will undoubtedly be found amusing by a student in 2085. A recent example is the following. A current study on Type A and B behavior individuals refutes the results of earlier findings. Does one blame the individual for having changed from Type A behavior to Type B behavior to now finding out (for the present time) that he should have stayed with the former behavior? Or relating back to Milio, does the individual, on a daily basis, have the time, money, energy, to implement all the wellness behaviors one should? How do all individuals keep informed of all wellness behaviors? The concern with distributive justice, mentioned earlier in this paper, relates to this latter question. Individuals, for a host of reasons (education, income, etc.) have varying degrees of accessibility to information about wellness. Thus, the concern about distributive justice. Besides the first concern of a changing body of knowledge, there is also the aspect of changing rules in a society. The Simontons emphasize the point in their care of cancer patients that there is a difference between being "to blame" for something and having "participated" in it. "It makes no sense to blame persons living in this society for becoming ill in light of the rules they were taught for dealing with their emotions and feelings. Few individuals in our culture have been taught how to deal with emotions and feelings appropriately" (Simonton, 1981, p. 105). Other examples of how societal rules have changed include attitudes and actions surrounding cigarette smoking and alcohol ingestion. During World War II, cigarettes were disbursed freely to men in the Armed Services. Now, there are numerous programs, policies, etc., that promote smoking cessation. There are policies that provide financial penalties for the smoker and financial incentives for the nonsmoker. Reduced cost of alcoholic drinks at Officer's Clubs at military bases, "twofers" at bars, etc., are examples of an earlier societal milieu that is now changing. There are many more examples that could be given of changing bodies of knowledge or the changing rules of a society -- but, the impact of these has to be acknowledged before one would blame the victim.

A common thread for many authors who articulate their concern about victim blaming is the need to be aware of the paradigm one is using for problem identification and problem solving. For example, one could argue at the present time, that many wellness advocates are using a medical model of disease causation versus a biopsychosocial model of causation and that undue emphasis is being put on one aspect of the public health triad -- the host. Others would identify the problems differently by using a biopsychosocial model of causation and by placing equal emphasis on two parts of the triad -- environment and host. Many authors have spoken to the need for changes in macro structures which would make it easier for the individual to choose and practice wellness behaviors. An historical example that is pertinent will be discussed. "As Dubos has shown, the great advances in health in the eighteenth and nineteenth centuries were largely the result of social reforms that alleviated some of the pollution, dirt, poor housing, crowding, and malnutrition that had come from the industrial revolution. And although it is generally taken for granted that the introduction of antibiotics and effective immunization campaigns

65

were the key determining factors in the success of the fight against infectious diseases, Powles and McKeown provide convincing evidence to the contrary". "To be clear, immunization and antibiotics certainly are effective means to intervene in individuals and they have contributed to the almost total elimination of infectious diseases in advanced industrialized societies. The point is that resources have been invested for infectious diseases under the belief that immunization and antibiotics were the central causes of the diminution of mortality and morbidity from infections, while changes in the larger environment were, in fact, the prime causal factors" (Renaud, 1978, 103-105).

Other authors have analyzed that the incidence of certain communicable diseases was decreasing at the historical time when immunizations were being discovered and used. Some authors have cited the decreasing virulence of the organisms at this same time period. Other research points to the correlation of an increasing food supply and the decreasing incidence of communicable diseases. There are implications from such historical examples that could be applied to the wellness movement today in terms of problem solving at the macro level, i.e., putting emphasis on the environmental third of that public health triad. For example, many communicable and infectious diseases were prevented because of macro structures in society, e.g., engineering practices, health department sanitation policies, etc., that resulted in safe water, food, and milk supplies. In essence, individuals benefitted from environmental manipulation. They were able to prevent illness without expending energy on daily habits of choice. Thus when comparing and contrasting earlier time periods to the present, it can be seen that communicable and infectious diseases weren't conquered by individual effort alone, i.e., immunizations and antibiotics. Rather, macro structures -- both private and public sectors, i.e., the environmental leg of the triad -- was as important, if not more so, for the changing statistics.

From this author's perspective, the real challenge for the wellness movement is to identify those structures to change or initiate that will provide the individual with ease in choosing and practicing wellness behaviors. Allen is one theorist who is studying a cultural change model for promoting wellness.

Concern about being more oriented to macro structures is also voiced by those who are concerned that the wellness movement is too individual-oriented. One can't have a well individual in an unwell family, community, country, or world. Yet the emphasis predominantly is on individual activities and outcomes. Some have analyzed this as perhaps a by-product of the "me" decade of the 1970's or the "Yuppie" movement of the 1980's. Further observation is that the wellness movement is definitely a white middle-class phenomenon (Allegrante and Green, 1981). Other authors have noted that the self-responsibility concept of the wellness movement relates well to one U.S. ideological principle -- "pull yourself up by your bootstraps." While this principle is widely held by many Americans, its promise of the "better life" is illusory for many. The concerns mentioned here have direct implications for victim blaming and distributive justice. Davis has warned of "creeping elitism" in the wellness movement. He is concerned about the tendency to ignore those who due to social circumstances and/or government policies can neither avoid health hazards nor afford the self-care measures necessary to deal with them.

Several authors have addressed the need to look at a macro paradigm for causation and problem solving. Dubos has written, "Health and disease are the expressions of the relative degree of success or failure experienced by man as he tries to respond adaptively to environmental challenges, and also to the inner demands created in him by traditions and aspirations... Many, if not most chronic disorders are the secondary and delayed consequences of adaptive responses that were useful at first, but are faulty in the long run" (Renaud, 1978, 105). He continues by making the point that many diseases are because of a capitalist industrial model -- not necessarily age-related degenerative. Renaud speaks to similar concepts, "To the new diseases engendered by capitalist industrial growth, such as ischemic heart disease, various cancers, and mental and nervous disorders, medicine has evolved an approach which is incapable of acting upon the social component of the etiology of diseases" (Renaud, 1978, 103). Zola has written, "C.S. Lewis warned us more than a quarter of a century ago that "man's power over nature is really the power of some men over other men, with nature as their instrument. By locating the source and the treatment of problems in an individual, *other levels of interventions are effectively closed* (italics mine)" (Zola, 1978, 95).

McKinlay writes, "Individuals are either doing something that they ought not to be doing, or they are not doing something that they ought to be doing. If only they would recognize their individual culpability and alter their behavior in some appropriate fashion, they would improve their health status or the likelihood of not developing certain pathologies. To use the upstream-downstream analogy, one could argue that people are blamed (and, in a sense, even punished) for not being able to swim after they, perhaps against their own volition, have been pushed into the river by the manufacturers of illness" (Renaud, 1978, 117).

Crawford echoes concerns as above but also raises the point that the complexity and bureaucratization of our society diminishes the power of the individual (Crawford, 1977). Such an argument speaks to the lack of power that individuals, as individuals, have over hazardous working conditions, environmental conditions, etc. -- all of which contribute to the chronic illnesses. Of significance to those who attempt to remedy such toxic hazards is the outcome of the employee who pursued the hazards of Agent Orange for servicemen -- she was fired. Shapiro and Shapiro have also written about such concerns. They analyze that the wellness movement may merge with humanism in such a way as to cause victim blaming (Shapiro, 1979). They speak not only to social causation of disease but address frontally the marketing industry and profit that is made by same. "A great deal of energy, brain power, and above all, money has gone into marketing bad health in this

68

country... If the individual alone is responsible for his or her own well-being, society can encourage us to abuse our bodies and, even worse, can continue to profit from those abuses" (1979, 211).

Although there is merit to wellness behaviors, Illich has observed that the antagonistic relationship between the individual and disease is uniquely Western (Illich, 1976). An application of Kluckholn's theory would also support this. Other cultures see disease and death as part of life and are more accepting of both. This model of man as conqueror is not as present with them. He speaks to the irony that we have come full circle -- however, now we put the omnipotence in health care not on the physician-- but on the individual. There is a myth that if only one could control enough, or be disciplined enough, one could prevent illness and death. Gonzalez has also written about the present tendency of science and technology to have an inversion of priorities, i.e., to have power over the universe rather than knowledge of it (Gonzalez, 1 979). When looking at the model for self-responsibility, it is important to keep in mind that the model falls within the purview of this larger anthropological analysis.

Lessor is another author who is concerned about victim blaming when the main culprit may be working conditions. "If one has only to improve one's 'fitness' or 'knowledge' the implication is that the problem begins and ends with the individual" (1984, 147). She agrees with the point that how we solve a problem is dependent on the paradigm we use for viewing its causation. She cites examples of occupational hazards.

Pilisuk has written on the correlation of social support network to indices of morbidity (Pilisuk, 1982). There is an inverse relationship.

In our society, the forces of careerism, autonomy, mobility, privacy, and achievement tend to disrupt our traditional roots and ties and make difficult the continuity of new bonds. This is a societal change and phenomenon that mitigates against wellness, but again is another societal causation factor that must be considered before blaming someone for his illness.

Issues related to distributive justice have been raised throughout this paper. Salmon writes, "Given these redirections, it appears that the invisible hand of the marketplace responds more to profit opportunities than to people's health needs" (Salmon, 1983, 131). Although he is talking about other parts of the health system, I believe there are analogies to the wellness sector. He continues, "the competition proponents envision the health care market as a place for people with money to enter and buy services; this includes middle and upper income groups who can afford them..." (p. 132). As mentioned earlier, thus far the wellness movement is predominantly a middle-class phenomenon. On an individual basis, some individual may wish to practice wellness behaviors but not have the disposable income to join programs, etc., that others can with little pain or sacrifice to their family budget. At the work level, some companies may have programs that are noninclusive for all employees. Thus, the issues raised by the distributive justice dilemma mitigate against victim blaming.

In summary, it is important that this paper not be read as an acceptance, rationalization, tolerance, or condoning of illness behaviors. Rather, this author is firmly committed to promotion of wellness behaviors and also believes that most individuals are also committed to that and to doing what is in their best interest. But, as this paper has articulated, there are barriers and reasons that exist that keep people from doing so. The challenge for health care providers and societal policy makers is finding not only individual but, more importantly, macro structures that will facilitate the maximization of wellness behaviors. Until that occurs, the author is concerned that the cost containment era and the "monetization of all values" will promote a victim blaming ideology. R. Buckminister Fuller summarizes this author's analysis best, "I had decided in 1927 that there were two things you could do if you wanted to improve the total existence of man on earth. You could try to reform man himself or you could reform the environment, and the environment, if properly reformed, would allow man to really behave well. I don't think I can improve on man" (Hirsh, 1981).

REFERENCES

1. Allegrante, J.P. and Green, L.W. (1981). "When Health Policy Becomes Victim Blaming." *New England Journal of Medicine.* 305(25), 1528-1529.
2. Archer, S.A. and Fleshman, R.P. (1985). *Community Health Nursing* (Monterey, California: Wadsworth Health Sciences).
3. Ardell, D.B. (1977). *High Level Wellness* (Emmaus, PA: Rodale Press).
4. Blattner, B. (1981). *Holistic Nursing* (Englewood Cliffs, New Jersey: Prentice-Hall).
5. Bordieri, J.E., Salodky, M.L., and Mikos, K.A. (1985). "Physical Attractiveness and Nurses' Perceptions of Pediatric Patients." *Nursing Research,* 34(1), 24-26.
6. Campbell, J. and Humphreys, J. (1984). *Nursing Care of Victims of Family Violence* (Reston, Virginia: Reston Publishing).
7. Connelly, C.E. (1984). "Economic and Ethical Issues in Patient Compliance." *Nursing Economics,* 2, 342-347.
8. Crawford, R. (1977). "You Are Dangerous to Your Health: The Ideology and Politics of Victim Blaming." *International Journal of Health Services,* 7(4), 663-680.
9. Dracup, K.A. and Mileis, A.I. (1982). "Compliance: An Interactionist Approach." *Nursing Research,* 31(1), 31-35.
10. Fielding, J.E. and Breslow, L. (1983). "Health Promotion Programs Sponsored by California Employers." *American Journal of Public Health,* 73(5), 538-542.
11. Flynn, P.A. (1980). *Holistic Health* (Bowie, MD: Prentice-Hall).
12. Geller, J. and Butler, K. (1981). "Study of Educational Deficits as the Cause of Hospital Admission for Diabetes Mellitus in a Community Hospital." *Diabetes Care,* 4(4), 487-489.
13. Gochman, D.S. (1974). "Preventive Encounters and Their Psychological Correlates." *American Journal of Public Health,* 64(11), 1096-1097.
14. Gonzalez, S.P. (1979). "Bioethics and the Oc-

cupational Health Nurse." *Occupational Health Nursing,* September, 11-15.
15. Hallal, J.C. (1982). "The Relationship of Health Beliefs, Health Locus of Control, and Self Concept to the Practice of Breast Self-Examination in Adult Women." *Nursing Research,* 31(3), 137+.
16. Hirsh, J. and Hannock, L. (1981). *Mosby's Manual of Clinical Nursing Procedures* (St. Louis: C.V. Mosby).
17. Hochbaum, G.M. (1982). "Certain Problems in Evaluating Health Education." *Health Values: Achieving High Level Wellness.* 6(1), 14-20.
18. Iglehart, J.K. (1982). "Health Care and American Business." *New England Journal of Medicine,* 306(2), 120-124.
19. Iglehart, J.K. (1984). "Smoking and Public Policy." *New England Journal of Medicine,* 310(8), 539-544.
20. Illich, I. (1976). *Medical Nemesis* (New York: Pantheon).
21. Laufman, L. and Weinstein, J. (1978). "Values and Prevention." *Health Values: Achieving High Level Wellness,* 2(5), 270-273.
22. Laughlin, J.A. (1982). "Wellness at Work: A Seven Step 'Dollars and Sense' Approach." *Occupational Health Nursing,* November, 9-13.
23. Lee, J.S., Rom, W.N., and Craft, B.F. (1983). "Preventing Disease and Injury in the Work Place: Issues and Solutions." *Family and Community Health,* May, 1-10.
24. Lessor, R. (1984). "Occupational Health Policy: Addressing Personal Troubles or Social Problems?" *Occupational Health Nursing.* March, 146-150.
25. Lowery, B.J. and DuCette, J.P. (1976). "Disease-Related Learning and Disease Control in Diabetes as a Function of Locus of Control." *Nursing Research.* 25(5), 358-362.
26. Milio, N. (1981). *Promoting Health through Public Policy* (Philadelphia: F.A. Davis).
27. Murphy, M.M. (1982). "Why Won't They Shape Up? Resistance to the Promotion of Health." *Canadian Journal of Public Health,* 73, 427-430.

28. Navarro, V. (1976). *Medicine Under Capitalism* (New York: Prodist).

29. O'Donnell, M.P. and Ainsworth, P. (1984). *Health Promotion in the Workplace* New York: John Wiley and Sons).

30. Pellegrino, E. (1983, Summer). Seminar Presentation, NEH Institute -- Health Care Ethics for Health Faculty, Lexington, Kentucky: University of Kentucky.

31. Pender, N.J. (1975). "A Conceptual Model for Preventive Health Behavior." *Nursing Outlook,* 23(6), 385-390.

32. Pilisuk, M. (1982). "Delivery of Social Support: The Social Inoculation." *American Journal of Orthopsychiatry.* 52(1), 20-31.

33. Polin, W. and Ravenholt, R.T. (1984). "Tobacco Addiction and Tobacco Mortality." *Journal of American Medical Association,* 252:20, 2849-2854.

34. Renaud, M. (1978). "On the Structural Constraints to State Intervention in Health." In J. Ehrenriech (Ed.), *The Cultural Crisis of Modern Medicine,* pp. 101-120 (New York: Monthly Review Press).

35. Salmon, J.W. (1983). "Who Benefits from Competition in Health Care?" *Nursing Economics,* 1, 129-134.

36. Shapiro, J. and Shapiro, D.H. (1979). "The Psychology of Responsibility -- Some Second Thoughts on Holistic Medicine." *New England Journal of Medicine,* 301(4), 211-212.

37. Sidel, V.W. (1979). "Public Health in International Perspective: From 'Helping the Victim' to 'Blaming the Victim' to 'Organizing the Victim.' *Canadian Journal of Public Health,* 70(4), 234-239.

38. Simonton, O.C., Matthews-Simonton, S., Creighton, J.L. (1981). *Getting Well Again* (New York: Bantam).

39. Stanhope, M. and Lancaster, J. (1984). *Community Health Nursing.* (St. Louis: C.V. Mosby Co.).

40. Steckel, S.B. and Swain, M.A. (1977). "Contracting with Patients to Improve Compliance." *Hospitals,* 51, 81-84.

41. Taylor, R. and Thoma, K. (1985). "Mortality Patterns in the Modernized Pacific Island Nation of Nauru." *American Journal of Public Health*, 75(2), 149-155.
42. Vanderhaar, G.A. (1985). "The Making of Enemies." *Pax Christi USA*. March, 7-9.
43. Wilner, D.M., Walkley, R.P. and Goerke, L.S. (1973). *Introduction to Public Health* (New York: MacMillan).
44. Wilson, H.S. and Kneisl, C.R. (1979). *Psychiatric Nursing* (Menlo Park, California: Addison-Wesley Co.).
45. Zola, I.K. (1978). "Medicine as an Institution of Social Control." In J. Ehrenriech (Ed.), *The Cultural Crisis of Modern Medicine*, 80-100. (New York: Monthly Review Press).

WELLNESS AND JUSTICE
Commentary on Professor Furlong

By William F. Finn, M.D.

It has been a delight to hear the comprehensive and thoughtful analysis of the wellness movement which Professor Furlong has given us this morning.

It intrigues me that she has not provided a definition of wellness or told us whether she equates wellness with health. Even though it is imperfect, I have used the definition of health propounded by the Word Health Organization in 1946, "Health is the state of complete physical, mental and social wellbeing and not merely the absence of disease or infirmity." I have regarded health and wellness as roughly equivalent, feeling that wellness is perhaps a more positive state, something like health plus.

Dr. Furlong recounts some benefits of the wellness movement:

First, reduction in morbidity and mortality. While this is certainly true, is it due to the wellness movement or is it due to public health measures-- sanitation, pure water, etc. ?

Second, she alleges a decrease in health costs, but public analyses and private experience question this. New drugs, new procedures and new machines increase the cost of health care.

Third, she mentions health status indications which can be questioned when presented on a purely statistical basis. It is easy to measure disease prevention, but almost impossible to ascertain health promotion.

Fourth, she states there is an increase in economic productivity. This is equivalent to regarding human health as being determined by the Gross National Product. Man the human being is viewed only as Man the worker.

Lastly, she refers to an increase in the potential of the individual. While this may be true, it is virtually impossible to prove.

I agree completely with Dr. Furlong as she traces the causation of disease from the agent (bacterium or virus), to the environment, and finally to 1987, where man is the primary cause. Changes in the illness and death rates which we see now are due to the elimination of communicable and infectious diseases and their replacement by diseases associated with the aging process and the individual's pattern of living.

Dr. Furlong has selected three ethical issues for more detailed discussion:

1. Paternalism and Autonomy;
2. Distributive justice; and
3. Blaming the victim.

Paternalism and Autonomy are traditional opponents. The apparent differences between them were highlighted by the increased advocacy of patients' rights a decade ago. But are truly the autonomy of patients and the paternalistic attitudes of physicians the true adversaries? Are not the true opponents the welfare of self and the welfare of others? Must not the welfare of self be restricted to prevent infringement on the rights of others? At times the judgement of Solomon is necessary to achieve the just balance. Is not a benign paternalism dedicated to trying to modify a patient's behavior for his own betterment in the patient's best interest? Can a physician stand by impartially when actions of a patient are likely to harm himself or others?

Her second ethical concern, distributive justice, is shared by all of us. Her statement, "The real challenge for the wellness movement is to identify those structures to change or initiate that will provide the individual with ease in choosing and practicing wellness behaviors," could well be used as a battle cry for the wellness movement. But it is much easier to state it than to effect it and to maintain it. Who should decide what plan to use and, if it is not effective, to change it? It must be flexible, changing with the body of knowledge and the rules of society. But how to correct differences in education or even more fundamentally, in literacy? How to provide economic opportunity for upward social and financial mobility? Obviously, while it should be across the board, more opportunity should be provided for the sick, the poor, and those with lesser degree of education. Yet Professor Furlong tells us that wellness is a white, middle class movement. She further states that some corporations which practice it as a business policy restrict it to the upper levels of management. But to be truly just, it should be available to all levels of employees and, on a broader societal scale, should provide the opportunity to all people.

Dr. Furlong devotes the balance of her concern to the third ethical issue, "blaming the victim." She has said, "victim blaming with the wellness movement could be a short term remedy for anxious concerns about escalating health care costs." While this may contribute to the mental attitude of blaming the victim, the issues is much more fundamental. The question is whether the individual is responsible for his health status and if he is not, who is? Is it the obligation of the healing professions? Society? The government? Or in most instances does it come right down to the patient himself or the more euphemistic term "the victim?"

What is the individual's duty to initiate his health care and to maintain it by behaviors which promote wellness? There is no question that the patient can be regarded as a victim when there are genetic or congenital impairments, when disease is due to environmental injuries or infections, and also when disease is caused by a true accident which has not been caused by the negligence of the patient. It is also true that society and government should contribute to public health measures and other macro-systems to promote wellness. These can provide opportunities for health inducing environments as well as disseminating information. Here the problem of distributive justice arise again.

But is the patient always a victim? Let us consider some diseases. To name a few:

1. Sexually transmitted diseases.
2. Unplanned pregnancy.
3. Obesity.
4. Emphysema.
5. Cancer of the lungs, mouth, or tongue.

6. Delirium tremens, and the
7. Effects of ingestion of addictive drugs (e.g., cocaine and marijuana).

Now let us consider some activities:

1. Driving when drunk.
2. Sky diving.
3. Refusal to wear a helmet when motor-cycling.
4. Drag racing.
5. Downhill skiing.
6. Failure to buckle seat belts, and
7. Non-compliance with diet -- both with respect to calories and food selection.

Now a few occupations:

1. Working in an asbestos or radium factory.
2. Test piloting, and
3. Newspaper reporting in a war zone.

All of these activities and occupations as well as many others can be viewed as life in the fast lane or even as a form of chronic suicide.

Let us think of the effects of cigarette smoking. Cancer of the lung, larynx and esophagus is increased 7 to 15 times, cancer of bladder, kidney and prostate are doubled. Emphysema and chronic obstructive pulmonary diseases are increased 10 to 20 times.

There are an estimated 10 to 15 million alcoholics in the United States, the annual cost in 1982 was twelve billion dollars and now is higher, so that it almost approximates the 1987 federal deficit. While it is true some of the patients afflicted with the above diseases are victims, the vast majority of these diseases are self-caused.

Professor Furlong inquires, "Is a blaming-the-victim mentality antithetical to the healing relationship between provider and patient?" It can be if the physician, nurse, or therapist adopts an "Oh! You Poor Dear" attitude when the illness is due to the patient's voluntary lack of compliance, omission or commission. I have always had better and more permanent results by asking non-judgmental questions like, "Why do you expose yourself like this?" It is paradoxical to expect to exercise autonomy without accepting responsibility. Patient non-compliance, at times bordering on recidivism, should not be fostered, but should be resisted in a rational, dedicated, and concerned manner.

I agree completely with Professor Furlong on the issues of distributive justice. Like her, I believe that the wellness movement is too orientated to the individual. But then were else can it begin and where else can it be maintained? The wellness movement at the present time overstresses the physical aspects of health and does not lay enough emphasis on the emotional and metal components of man's nature. Like the ancients, I subscribe to modifications of the movement which would aim toward a sound mind in a sound body. Dr. Furlong and I while we agree on most of the basics, differ on the so-called "blaming the victim" attitude. I condone it less and feel that the patient is not always the victim and when he is not, he should change his attitudes and habits to cooperate in an active fashion with nursing and medical advisors in the efforts to correct his illness and to maintain his health in the future.

THE ART OF ACUPUNCTURE AND AN ETHICS OF HEALING

By John G. Sullivan
Elon College

Part I: *The Art of Acupuncture*

Acupuncture(1) is a primary health care modality which has flourished in China for more than twenty-five centuries. What is new for us in the United States is itself an ancient healing art. Given its long history, acupuncture is hardly "experimental" in the sense of untried; "it is no more experimental as a mode of medical treatment than is the Chinese language as a mode of communication."(2) Further-more, unlike other practices (e.g. blood letting) which have not survived the advent of Western scientific medicine, acupuncture is a healing mode which exists in complementarity with Western practices in countries such as China where it is amply appreciated.

These remarks are a caveat against cultural bias and an invitation to take acupuncture seriously. It is my contention that as we come to understand acupuncture more fully, it will provide an opportunity to expand our understanding of the whole area of health and healing. Acupuncture is specially suited to provide this bridge because it is both very close to and very distant from the standard Western medical model.

On the one hand, acupuncture stands close to our Western sense of reality. It lays claim to a technology of intervention (e.g., needles, moxibustion) which is undergirded by sophisticated theoretical models (e.g. points, meridians, principles of energetic balancing) and which produces manifest changes in the physical body.

It is not surprising that we are especially impressed by physical results. When Western physi-cians and journalists accompanied President Nixon to China in February of 1972, they witnessed surgery being performed with acupuncture needles used for anesthetics. When the United States District Court

80

for Southern Texas had to assure itself that acupuncture done by skilled practitioners was safe and effective, it relied on a mass of testimony and concluded that acupuncture does indeed work. Interestingly, the court assembled photographic documentation showing the successful use, in veterinary medicine, of acupuncture on animals; it took that as evidence against the view that acupuncture works on the so-called "placebo" effect.

What the U.S. District Court concluded is best stated in its own words: "Whatever the best explanation is for how acupuncture works, one thing is clear: it does work. All the evidence put before the court indicates that, when administered by a skilled practitioner for certain types of pain and dysfunction, acupuncture is both safe and effective."(3)

I shall return to this important statement later. For the moment, I want simply to point out that acupuncture and allopathic medicine both seek explainable changes on the plane of physical reality. Insertion of needles is a physical intervention. Acupuncture claims that shifts in the energy field ("*ch'i*") occur as a result of such interventions and these shifts are not dependent on the belief state of the patient. Crudely put, one no more has to "believe in" acupuncture for results to occur than one has to "believe in" Western medicine for results to occur. Acupuncture does depend on a subtle set of diagnostic skills -- traditionally named: "to see, to hear, to ask, to feel." But acupuncture is not simply a "talking cure;" in addition to speaking and listening, there are also the insertion of needles, the maps of bioenergetics, the shifts experienced in the physical body. Insofar as both acupuncture and allopathic medicine intervene directly at a physical level, both share an anchor to a common terrain -- physical reality/physical change.

On the other hand, acupuncture is immensely dissimilar to Western medicine. It is ancient rather than modern, Eastern rather than Western. Initially, a Westerner seeking to understand acupuncture on its own terms encounters a language, a set of notions and a world view which are unfamiliar and strange. The *Huang Ti Nei Ching* or Yellow Emperor's *Classic of Internal Medicine* (dated c. 200 B.C.) is acknowledged as foundational by all schools of acupuncture. But to understand this work, one must understand such notions as the Tao, Ch'i (or Qi) energy, and Yin-Yang dynamics. These and other notions define the context of acupuncture, and herein lies a special difficulty. Acupuncture exists within one total interpretive context; Western medicine, within another. To speak of an organ, say the heart, will have one sense in the allopathic paradigm and quite another in the acupuncture paradigm. To speak of a symptom (or even of health itself) will have one set of implications in the allopathic paradigm and another in the acupuncture paradigm.

Confronted with the aspect of difference or otherness, one may bemoan the difficulties or celebrate the diversity. I wish to stress "otherness as opportunity." To this end, I point out five differences between acupuncture and allopathic medicine.

> *1.   The   Energetic   Field: Patterns   rather   than parts.*

In acupuncture, the focus of treatment is on the energetic field within which the patient and practitioner exist. The contrast here is with an allopathic view that the isolated person (autonomous, atomistic, bounded by the skin) is the subject of treatment. Such a Western view, while uncongenial to those doing family counselling or engaged in public health projects, still runs deep.(4) The paradigm of acupuncture recognizes an objective pattern of nature, including human nature. It acknowledges "the pattern that connects" and calls it TAO. It speaks of patterns of *ch'i* energy within the body and between the organism and environment. The healing principles and techniques of acupuncture affect the flow and intensity of ch'i energy. The focus on the energetic field -- on pattern rather than isolated parts -- is distinctive of acupuncture.

> *2.   The   Vertical   Axis: Multi-rather   than mono-leveled reality.*

The ancient viewpoint of macrocosm-microcosm sees reality as multi-dimensional. Persons-in-the-world are perceived as operating within and across levels of bodily, emotional, intellectual, and spiritual interchange. The dimensions are many; as a shorthand, we refer to the manifold as the three dimensions of body-mind-spirit. Diagnosis in traditional acupuncture involves attention to color, sound, odor, emotion, to story and season, time of day and time of life, daytime behaviors and nighttime dreams. The dream is taken as seriously as the backache; dryness of spirit is as significant as dryness of the tongue. In the Western view, such levels (where acknowledged) are assigned to different specialists -- the medical doctor, the psychologist, the spiritual director, etc.

3.   *Goal of treatment: Ideal as present vs. ideal as future.*

Energetic field and vertical axis are features which define the acupuncture context. The third feature looks to how the goal of treatment is conceptualized.

In the West, the ideal is seen as what is not yet, what is in the future, what will be if and when it is actualized. The image of ideal as future suggests that what exists now is imperfect, is non-ideal. Thus, we have a split between "is" and "ought." What "is" becomes the real world; what "ought to be" becomes the ideal (the "unreal" world). The image of ideal as future also suggests that change involves effort, striving, perhaps even competition for scarce rewards.

In the East, we are not confronted with "is" versus "ought." The ideal is what is and the defect is what is -- but on different levels. The ideal is how things are at their depth, when seen in their fullness. The defect is how things are when understanding is restricted to the surface. Notice that under this formulation, the ideal is already and always present beneath or beyond the surface illusions. Here the ideal IS the real. What I take myself to be (my identification with the content of my life) is not what

I truly am at my depth (where I am at one with the context of my life). On such an understanding, going from defect to ideal is more like waking up than making New Year's resolutions, more like letting go of obstacles and illusory identifications than striving for what one does not have. At the surface level, there is disharmony; at the depth, one has never been other than what one was meant to be.

The dualism of surface vs. depth is provisional. Indeed, the East aims ultimately at a mode of understanding which is non-dualistic. This brings us to the fourth feature: the nature of change.

4. *Dynamics of Change: "Both-and" rather than "either-or".*

Where a pre-Socratic philosopher like Heraclitus saw movement as a clash of opposites, his Chinese counterparts spoke of yin-yang as a harmony of opposites -- as arising together, as equally necessary, as unfolding according to natural rhythms. In the Yin-Yang approach to balancing opposites, polarities exist, but they are not thought of in "either-or" fashion nor judged as "negative-positive."

The Chinese ideogram for "crisis" is composed of the character for "danger" and the character for "opportunity". In situations that we label positive, there are dangers; in situations that we label negative, there are opportunities. This approach to polarity as paradox has implications for healing.

The paradox is this: when humans are convinced that they are alright just as they are -- then they can change. In other words, we can let go of surface identities if we experience a deeper center and source of worth. We are BOTH our imbalances AND our core wholeness.

In acupuncture, even the underlying imbalance is not viewed simplistically. It is both imbalance insofar as energy is blocked and opportunity insofar as energy unblocked is a powerful source of re-vision, recovery and renewal.

5. *Metaphoric rather than literal language.*

Thus far, I have mentioned four features: energetics, reality as multi-leveled, the ideal as present and change as embracing "both-and" dialectics. The fifth feature concerns language. Acupuncture arose in a place (China) where language was pictorial, and at a time when people lived close to nature. Where nature (including human nature) is seen as multi-dimensional, it makes sense to prefer a language which is also multi-dimensional. Acupuncture, arising in this world view, framed its models in metaphoric language, rooted in the processes of nature. Thus, the Law of the Five Elements speaks of water, wood, fire, earth, and metal. And it correlates each of these with a season, an emotion, a color, and much more. The encouragement of associational thinking allows connections to be made among the levels of body-mind-spirit. Furthermore, use of poetic, non-technical language allows patient and practitioner to communicate in rich and healing ways. Such imagistic discourse gives patients ways to imagine who they are and what is going on with them.

With this mention of language, I conclude discussion of the art of acupuncture -- how it is similar and dissimilar to Western medicine. In the second part of my presentation, I turn to consider an ethics of healing.

Part II: *An Ethics of Healing*

There is a fundamental baseline for any ethics of the healing professions. The dictum derives from the Hippocratic Oath. It persists in its Latin form: "Primum non nocere," which we may translate as "First and foremost, cause no harm." More recently, it has been said: "The one thing a hospital should NOT do is spread disease." That, I take it, is no simple task.(5) Simple or not, safety is a prime ethical imperative. Furthermore, in addition to causing no harm, it is hoped that treatment will do some good. Hence, there is the further directive that treatment be, up to some agreed standard, effective. This dual standard of safety and effectiveness is a desideratum in any health-care modality. In the case of acupuncture, the above-quoted Texas District Court spoke with admirable clarity about the assurance sought: "All the evidence put before the court indicates that, when administered by a skilled practitioner for certain types of pain and dysfunction, acupuncture is both safe and effective."

While I concur with the verdict of the court, I present no independent brief. Such a venture would go well beyond the scope of this paper.(6) I do emphasize that the court is exactly correct to stress the importance of the four elements noted, namely, (1) practitioner skill, (2) safety, (3) effectiveness, and (4) range of intervention. In all that follows, I take it as given that acupuncture, properly done, is safe and effective for a range of imbalances.

A. *Informed Consent: An Exercise in Reframing*

In the first part of this paper, I tried to show that acupuncture -- as applied Eastern philosophy -- provides an alternate context to consider health and healing. In this second part, I suggest that an ethics of healing take as its model the nature of healing itself. But if this has merit, then to reconceive healing may well lead us to reconceive our ethics of healing and to reframe some of the notions in medical ethics.

As an exercise in reframing, I wish to consider the principle of informed consent. I focus on informed consent because it appears so central and, at least *prima facie*, so unproblematic in modern medical ethics.(7) Certainly, in making any serious decision, one would wish to know the problem, the recommended remedy with its costs, risks, benefits, and any alternatives with their cost, risks, benefits, etc. One would also want the space to choose without pressure, untoward influence, or fear of abandonment. I focus on informed consent because it might be thought that informed consent would pose exceptional problems for acupuncture (and, in fact, for any approach which claims to attend to the person in his or her multi-leveled reality).

The issue of informed consent is formulated from the standpoint of the patient -- the "one being done to". The earliest medical codes are formulated from the standpoint of the practitioner. In the West, the Hippocratic Oath still remains the model of high standards for the medical profession.(8) The oath is taken by practitioners, and deals first with a physician's relationships to his teachers and colleagues and then with his relationship to his patients. This oath and later codes focus on the interpersonal domain, on what Lawrence Kohlberg calls a stage three -- ideal role maintaining -- perspective.(9) By accepting the commitment embodied in the Hippocratic Oath, the practitioner vows to use medical skills for the well-being (not the harm) of those to be served. Canons of confidentiality and propriety (e.g. against taking sexual liberties) appear. But, in what might be initially surprising to a student of modern medical ethics, there is no analogue for the principle of informed consent, though such instruction could easily be set forth as a duty (or special virtue) of doctors.

Recent literature in Western medicine makes scant mention of any rules or duties for patients.(10) When, in 1973, the American Hospital Association speaks to this side of the role relationship, the association entitles their document a "Statement on a Patient's Bill of Rights."(11) Although the language of rights is immediately present, and although this document issues from an institution, the political and economic context one associates with modern discussions of option and welfare rights is strikingly absent.(12) The document focuses on the interpersonal level. A patient's right to information, to informed consent, and to refuse treatment are explicit in the document, being articles two, three, and four of a dozen articles.

If one sets side by side the Hippocratic Oath and the Statement on a Patient's Bill of Rights, the contrast is instructive. Seen in this context, talk of informed consent, which to us seems so natural a requirement, begins to appear differently. It appears to conflate two separate concerns: first, concern to assure the patient that what to do (the proposed treatment plan) is a responsible, humane course of action, and, second, concern that the decision regarding what to do would rest with the patient. These two concerns are separable: knowing the "best" treatment is one thing and deciding for oneself is another. One could decide but not for what is best; one could be given what was best and not decide for oneself. When this is revealed, informed consent shows its roots in individualism and in the modern value given to self-determination as a key feature of personhood.(13) From this angle, informed consent appears in the context of an anti-paternalist polemic. The antagonistic language of ensuring rights tends to obscure the deeper ideal of promoting a mutuality between doctor and patient, a co-responsibility for care and cure.

B. *Acupuncture and Informed Consent*

Given this context, it might be thought that acupuncture (and more generally, any alternative healing modality which aspires to caring for persons across the multi-levels of body-mind-spirit) would have special problems with the requirement for informed consent. The charge might run as follows:

There are difficulties enough in supplying the conditions of informed consent in allopathic medicine. Yet here the intervention is primarily physical and the paradigm of Western science, while not understood in depth by most patients, is at least a culturally familiar one. When body and mind are treated, as in psychotherapy, there are further complications. The alternative forms of psychotherapy are manifold. It is complex to present the distinctive forms of interventions employed by such and such a therapy, to explain their point and purpose, risks and benefits. Nor is it a simple task to give a patient a sense of the range of alternative treatments with their costs and benefits. But suppose that in addition to responding to the levels of body and mind, one also undertakes to be receptive to imbalances on the level of spirit. Consider explaining the spiritual journey, the modes of transformation, and the responsibility of increased awareness/compassion.

If this is the charge, and if one is centered in an ethic of obligations,(14) then one might think that one is adding domains, and extending one's commitments. The image is additive -- going from physical technique to teaching, from teaching to therapy, from therapy to spiritual guidance. An ethic where obligations result (solely or principally) from contract gives a particularly strong picture of this additive process with every increase of domain signalling the need for fuller competence and fuller commitment. If this is indeed what one is doing, then the ethic of technique (taking responsibility for physical consequences) would be supplemented by an ethic of teaching; the ethic of teaching would be supplemented by an ethic of therapy; the ethic of therapy would be supplemented by an ethic of spiritual direction. All of this, it might be thought, would increase the difficulties of providing the conditions of informed consent. Add to this a healing modality which arises from an ancient rather than modern, an Eastern rather than Western, paradigm, and it might seem that the requirements of informed consent would be insurmountable. Such, at any rate, might be the charge.

If, however, we move out from under the additive image, if we begin to operate from within the standpoint of acupuncture, the landscape changes. The charge I have outlined would be puzzling to those acupuncturists of my acquaintance; it would not fit their experience. Rather than force the fit, it might be worthwhile to hear another voice, to imagine another possibility.

C. *Acupuncture and the Opportunity for Reframing*

In Part I of this paper, I suggested five features of the acupuncture world view: (1) the focus on energetic field, (2) the vertical axis of multi-leveled reality, (3) the ideal as already present, (4) a dialectical (both-and) notion of change, and (5) the preference for multi-leveled (metaphoric) language, From within this perspective, the issue appears differently. First, the energetic field is the entry point for supporting health and healing. When this is the focus, the idea of promoting a mutuality between doctor and patient -- a co-responsibility for care and cure -- appears closer at hand. From an acupuncture world view, it is nature -- within and without -- which does the healing. Both the acupuncturist and the person who comes to treatment stand within this healing context seeking to let go of barriers to a fuller mode of living. There is profound assurance and healing power in an approach where the ground and goal of life is the source that both practitioner and patient come from and go to. When this is appreciated, worries about one-sidedness diminish.

Secondly, in the acupuncture view, both parties to the healing dynamic are complex, multi-dimensional beings. They bring all these dimensions to the treatment room whether practitioners or patients are prepared to recognize them or not. What is going on occurs within and between the parties on bodily, emotional, intellectual and spiritual levels. Thus, it is not a matter of adding to, but of recognizing, what is already there.

But perhaps the worry is less about acknowledging complexity and more about the dangers of indoctrination as more dimensions of the person are considered relevant. Unquestionably, abuses may occur. In the space available, I can only suggest that the remaining three features of acupuncture tend to minimize a tendency to indoctrinate.

These features are: the ideal as already present, a dialectical (both-and) notion of change, and the preference for multi-leveled (metaphoric) language.

When mind, heart and spirit are spoken of in an acupuncture context, the goal is not seen narrowly; in fact, it is not a goal to be striven for at all. We all share already in what is central. At the core, the person is whole and dwells in a basic goodness beyond duality. Again, the paradigm of "both-and" change encourages humility. The person who asks and the practitioner who accepts the invitation to partnership BOTH ARE AND ARE NOT in touch with that wellspring of health, wholeness, and holiness. Neither aggression nor arrogance is called for. The way of acupuncture encourages not striving but letting go, not excluding, but including more fully. The ideal as present, and the dialectic of "both-and" change, act as hedges against the type of indoctrination that can occur when the goal is taken too narrowly and the means are construed in an "either-or," win/lose fashion.

Finally, an open metaphoric language calls us to concrete realities without the limits of literalism. In acupuncture, such language encourages personal discovery of what is needed -- beyond warring polarities. Given the metaphoric language, the dictum: "Educate, treat, educate." is perhaps less difficult than what allopathic health education envisages. This is because acupuncture's own technical vocabulary remains poetic, metaphoric, imagistic. And, as poetry across the ages shows, all peoples resonate to fundamental images of birth, growth, fear, death, and the seasons of life. People can understand and indwell an imagistic language far more easily (and sanely) than they can try to live within a techno-logical, machine-based language.

Part III: *Concluding Remarks*

By way of summary, let me call to mind the structure of this presentation. I began by noting that, among what have been called "the other medi-cines," acupuncture is especially suited to enter conversation with modern Western medicine. Like Western medicine, it is a physical intervention that claims to produce physical change. Unlike Western medicine, it stresses energetics, multi-dimensionality, presentness, dialectical change, and metaphoric language. It was my suspicion that when healing is situated in such a different setting, then an ethics of healing must likewise be reconceptualized.

To do some testing, I proposed that we consider the principle of informed consent -- partly because it seemed relatively unproblematic in modern Western ethics and partly because I myself once thought that wholistic healing would have difficulty with the principle of informed consent. The project of considering consent brought back into the picture the five features I earlier outlined. What I think emerges

91

from this exercise in reframing is a strengthened conviction that an ethics appropriate to acupuncture will follow the model of healing itself and will speak an open, metaphorical language much like acupuncture.(15) Such a direction opens up new possibilities for ethics beyond the current triad of rules, rights, and responsibility ethics. But the exploration, though Eastern, need not be partisan.

Perhaps going East is simply completing a circle and coming home.(16) Perhaps what is being rediscovered is what true healers of diverse traditions have long known. As that recognition prompts us to reconsider what healing is, it will also cause us to language very differently what we point to when we seek an ethics of healing.

ENDNOTES

1. The story of acupuncture is complex. In this paper, I shall speak of acupuncture as it is taught at the Traditional Acupuncture Institute in Columbia, Maryland. This school derives from an acupuncture system taught by J.R. Worsley in England and stressing the Five Element/Twelve Official (rather than the Eight Principle) model. For information on this tradition, see Dianne M. Connelly, *Traditional Acupuncture: The Law of the Five Elements* (Columbia, Md.: Centre for Traditional Acupuncture, 1975). For a writer from the eight principle tradition, see Ted J. Kaptchuk, *The Web That Has No Weaver: Understanding Chinese Medicine* (New York: Congdon and Weed, 1983).

2. The point is made by the United States District Court for the Southern District of Texas in affirming the right of Americans to seek acupuncture (7-9-80/Civil Action No. H-77-999).

3. *Ibid.*

4. For a general critique of the individualistic bias, see Roberto Mangabeira Unger, *Knowledge and Politics* (New York: Free Press, 1975).

5. For a discussion of iatrogenic disease, see Ivan Illich, *Medical Nemesis: The Expropriation of Health* (New York: Pantheon Books, 1976).

6. For further information of these issues, see the following: Robert M. Duggan, "An Overview of Completed Research on Acupuncture," *The Journal of Traditional Acupuncture,* 2 (1978):43-59; Ronald E. Kotzch, "Acupuncture Today," *East West Journal* (Jan. 1986): 58-65; R. Prasaad Steiner, "Acupuncture Cultural Perspectives, Parts 1 and 2", *Post Graduate Medicine,* 74 (1983); Robert O. Becker and Gary Seldon, *The Body Electric: Electromagnetism and the Foundations of Life* (New York: William Morrow and Co., 1985); and Manfred Porkert, *Theoretical Foundations of Chinese Medicine* (Cambridge, Mass.: MIT Press, 1974).

7. For a general treatment of this issue, see Bernard Barber, *Informed Consent in Medical*

Therapy and Research (New Brunswick, N.J.: Rutgers University Press, 1980). Also see, e.g. John Arras and Robert Hunt, eds., *Ethical Issues in Modern Medicine,* 2nd ed. (Palo Alto, Cal.: Mayfield Publishing Company, 1983), section 3, pp. 85-102.

8.   The Hippocratic Oath can be found in many sources. See, e.g., Arras and Hunt, *op. cit.,* p.46.

9.   See Lawrence Kohlberg, *Essays on Moral Development,* Vol. 1: *The Philosophy of Moral Development: Moral Stages and the Idea of Justice* (San Francisco: Harper and Row, 1981).

10.   However, it has come to my attention that the initial code of the American Medical Association in the founding year of that organization (1847) does list duties of patients (e.g. to be honest and open with their physicians). For this information, I am indebted to Michael Meyer, who received the doctorate in philosophy from the University of North Carolina at Chapel Hill in 1987.

11.   American Hospital Association, *Statement on a Patient's Bill of Rights* (Chicago: The Association, 1973. For critical discussion, see Elsie L. Bandman and Bertram Bandman, eds., *Bioethics and Human Rights* (Boston: Little, Brown and Company, 1978), Topic IV, "Rights in and to Health Care", pp. 255-284

12.   The use of "rights language" in the patient-practitioner context is hardly unproblematic. See, e.g., John Ladd, "Legalism and Medical Ethics," reprinted in Arras and Hunt, *op. cit.,* pp.57-64. For more extensive discussion, see Elsie L. and Bertram Bandman, *op. cit.*

13.   One feels here the influence of the eighteenth century thinkers such as Rousseau and Kant. For a critique of modern ethics from the perspective of a more ancient, communal, virtue-centered ethics, see Alasdair MacIntyre, *After Virtue: A Study in Moral Theory* (Notre Dame: University of Notre Dame Press, 1981)

14.   For the partial nature of an ethics of obligations, see Bernard Williams, *Ethics and the*

Limits of Philosophy (Cambridge, Mass.: Harvard University Press, 1985), chapter 10.

15. The roots of an ethics of acupuncture lie, it seems to me, in Eastern philosophy, in the superior person of the *I Ching,* in the complementary dance of Taoist and Confucian teaching, and in the Buddhist teaching of the Eight-fold path in its Theravada, Mahayana, and Vajrayana cycles. One valuable modern text which does ethics in the spirit I am suggesting is Chogyam Trungpa's book, *Shambhala: The Sacred Path of the Warrior* (Boston: Shambhala Publications, 1984). For my own thinking on this larger issue, see my article "Ethics in a Five Phase Framework," in the Spring 1987 issue of *The Journal of Traditional Acupuncture.*

16. For a full discussion of healing as returning home, see Dianne M. Connelly's new book, *All Sickness is Homesickness* (Columbia, Md.: Centre for Traditional Acupuncture, 1987).

ACUPUNCTURE AND PROFESSIONAL ETHICS
Commentary on Sullivan

By Michael Brannigan
Mercy College

My initial remarks will consider what I believe
are some of the many valuable ideas and suggestions
offered by Professor Sullivan. First, his notion of
"otherness as opportunity" is a necessary starting
point in the comparative study of cultures. The
emphasis upon acupuncture as a feasible bridge for
inter-cultural dialogue is sound, laudable, and
counteracts the prevailing notion of otherness as
source of alienation. I commend Professor Sullivan in
his sincere effort to transcend and ameliorate the
intellectual antagonisms which often persist, and
which continue to be constant obstacles to genuine
dialogue.

Sullivan gives us a five-fold schema highlighting
specific differences between Western and Chinese
theoretical frameworks, that is, between acupuncture
and allopathic medicine. This can be a most useful
paradigm for differentiating between divergent world-
views. Yet this same paradigm can be further
extended to signify differing concepts as to the very
definition of "science" itself. Comparative studies
often depict this fundamental difference in terms of
thematic contrasts, for example, the dynamic versus
static world, or the emphasis upon concrete reality as
opposed to abstractions, or what is immediate to
experience versus what is mediated. His five-fold
schema can be demonstrated if one views Western
science in terms of its emphasis upon the isolation of
variables. In other words, the testing of hypotheses
often depends upon certain aspects being lifted out of
their context and altered. The assumption here can
be that of an atomistic universe, a collection of
encapsulated items. Sullivan strongly indicates that
the Chinese world-view counters this. Another point
of contrast implied by Sullivan is the *de jure* approach to science in the West. This has been a
product of Western philosophy since the Greeks in

terms of the penchant to generalize and formulate *laws* of nature; thus, the "ideal" can mistakenly assume more reality than the objects themselves. A further point seems to be the prevailing divergence in time-consciousness between West and East. Any difference in time-consciousness is certainly a factor which demands continued study. If a fundamental distinction in time-orientation does exist, then it is an obvious ground for major discrepancies in world-views. In any case, the five-point framework posited by Sullivan is a most useful one in addressing these basic contrasts. His analysis of language is especially instructive, that is, the distinction between suggestive versus dualistic language.

Due to such fundamental differences in world-views, notions of health are thereby effected. Sullivan suggests that a traditional Chinese mode of treatment, namely acupuncture, can be considered a necessary complement to what he perceives to be a one-sidedness in the typical Western view of health. His suggestion is most valuable. Diagnostic method-ology in Chinese medicine insists upon establishing the root of illness and not simply treating the particular symptom. The holistic diagnostic process (seeing, interviewing, auscultation/olfaction, palpation, etc.) directs itself toward treating the whole patient as person. Prevention is emphasized over intervention. Health depends, not only upon environment, genetics, and fate, but also upon life-style, thoughts, emotions, etc. of the individual.

In his section dealing with specific ethical concerns, Sullivan reinstates what I consider to be a most crucial balance in the discussion of patient welfare. That is, along with the language of "rights," the language of "duties," or "obligations" of the patient must be restored. In his meaningful analysis of informed consent, emphasizing the duties of patients seems to be a natural extension in view of the Chinese holistic framework for medicine. Since, for the Chinese, health depends upon life-style as well as other factors, then the patient does bear primary responsibility for his health. For the Chinese, health is more than the absence of observable pathology. This therefore entails a broader view of rights, duties, and roles, and Sullivan's stress upon the "co-responsibility" and "mutuality" of responsibility is a healthy and necessary complement to much of the current discussion on ethics in medicine which understates the duties of patients themselves while perhaps overstating the case for rights.

It appears as if the traditional Chinese perspective, with its paradigm of acupuncture, comes close to a more phenomenological orientation to illness. A phenomenological orientation entails consideration of the total context of the healing process, in contrast to a dualistic, one-sided, technical approach. Healing is not only a science, but acknowledged as an art. Sullivan's paper is immensely significant in focusing upon a traditional treatment mode with important ethical implications. Moreover, the reframing of the physician-patient scenario also broadens notions of human personhood as well as moral responsibility.

This next part of my response will focus upon particular questions I address to Professor Sullivan for elaboration and/or clarification. He seems to rule out the efficacy of the "placebo" effect in acupuncture. Yet, is this in keeping with its theoretical basis of mind-body synthesis? Does not Western medicine, to some extent, rely upon this as well? To rephrase my point, although "shifts" in the energy field (*ch'i*) may not be, strictly speaking, dependent upon belief states of the individual, may not belief states still remain as a significant factor in recovery? Could not the notion of "belief state" be broadened to include an explicit trust in the practitioner? This would indicate a relationality component to "belief state" and not simply a matter of content, or *what* one believes in.

Sullivan indicates that, "*prima facie*," informed consent appears to be unproblematic in the West. However, given our Aristotelian inheritance in Western philosophy, the issue of informed consent seems to be constantly problematic, especially in the context of medical-ethical theory. There are basically three primary components within informed consent: a) disclosure -- which must grapple with questions of just how much information is given, and how relevant; b) voluntariness -- which takes one into sensitive issues of "coercion" versus influence and the significance of both environmental and internal factors; c) competency -- which contains a plethora of disputed issues. Let me focus upon the complex issues surrounding competency. At first hand, one can define competency in terms of an understanding of issues, alternatives, risks, benefits, etc., yet any acceptable criteria need to be acceptable on several levels: legal, psychiatric, philosophical, and clinically applicable. In competency assessment, good clinical determination must balance different, and sometimes competing, values of rationality, beneficence, and autonomy. Furthermore, the sensitive issues of the role of emotions inordinately enter into the discussion, for example, the utilization of psychotic defenses which seem to impede an awareness of the situation. It may feasibly be argued that not every emotional disturbance constitutes incompetence. To what degree does the presence of anxiety, which would naturally accompany many serious decisions, make one less competent? The assessment of competency and determining whether mental or emotional elements compromises rational decision-making is not only a psychiatric judgement, but entails consideration of philosophic assumptions and attitudes. Given my remarks, I would be most interested in what Professor Sullivan means by indicating the "unproblematic" nature of informed consent.

Sullivan strikes a most sensitive chord when he cautions us concerning the possibility of "indoctrination" as a very significant factor in the perception of acupuncture. This pertains, not only to acupuncture, but to the many "foreign" Eastern modalities transplanted into Western soil. One fundamentally significant question which his provocative analysis raises is this: since a necessary ingredient of informed consent entails a proper understanding of diagnosis, treatment alternatives, risks, benefits, etc., does this "proper understanding" necessitate a *shared world-view*? If so, then the danger of indoctrination becomes more obvious. Yet a proper understanding may perhaps occur at differing levels, that is, a comprehending of the rationale for treatment may not demand a shared-belief system or philosophy. In light of this, he needs to clarify or elaborate more precisely the "dangers of indoctrination."

A much disputed question in East-West dialogue remains one of synthesis: there appear to be deep, underlying differences in world-views, in attitudes, philosophies, concepts of time, notions of science, ideas of scientific explanation, notions of what needs to be explained -- given these deep-rooted divergencies, what would be the nature of dialogue? Can dialogue take place? Some suggest that the marriage of acupuncture and allopathic medicine can occur, and I am, to a certain extent, in agreement. Yet can fundamental perspectives be synthesized? What would be the prospects for global dialogue in this respect?

In conclusion, I am compelled to reaffirm the value of Professor Sullivan's paper as another positive step in the understanding and necessary appreciation of a foreign, traditional mode of treatment which offers a valuable complement to treatment modalities here in the West. Acupuncture has, in the West, suffered wide misunderstanding, especially through its misaligned association with parapsychology and the "occult." Yet Sullivan demonstrates rather soundly that it is not contradictory to Western scientific medicine. His paper suggests the need to *confirm* the positive results of both systems, acupuncture and allopathic, and to alleviate the intellectual antagonisms which exist as obstacles to the fruitful dialogue which Sullivan aptly encourages.

ETHICS OF LIMITED KNOWLEDGE IN THE HEALING PROFESSIONS

By Michael D. Bayles
Florida State University

The argument of this paper is meant to include all the healing professions, but it focuses on independent practitioners other than physicians. By "independent practitioners" I mean persons who provide their own diagnosis and treatment without direct, detailed supervision. For example, nurses working in physicians' offices are not independent practitioners, but nurse practitioners and most nurse midwives are. Chiropractors, clinical social workers, and many acupuncturists fall into this category.

Before proceeding, I confess my limited knowledge of, and attitude towards, the health professions. Except for dental and eye examinations, I try to avoid dealing professionally with all health care professionals. Moreover, except for one or two occasions, I have not been personally treated by members of nonstandard health professions. My attitude is similar to that of the skeptical old man who was asked whether he believed in baptism. "Believe in it," he replied, "Hell, I've seen it done!"

Health Care Professions and Occupations

The term profession can be defined in various ways for different purposes. For present purposes, three characteristics are central -- the provision of an important service, the possession of special knowledge, and work autonomy.(1) All the health care occupations provide an important service, for they all minister to health, which is a basic value. The focus here is on professional knowledge. Certification and higher education are also often suggested as defining characteristics of a profession. Higher education is a source of professional knowledge, and certification usually depends on a test of such knowledge. However, the argument herein applies so long as a healing occupation claims special expertise, whether or not that knowledge requires certification or higher education.   Work   autonomy   relates   to   being   an independent practitioner.   One can have a degree of work autonomy and not be an independent practitioner, but one cannot be an independent practitioner and lack work autonomy.

Two   other   distinctions   between   and   within professions must be noted.   One can roughly distinguish between professions that serve individual clients and those that serve large groups.   Among the latter are journalists and most engineers.   Most health care providers serve individuals, and many codes place the well-being of individual clients first.(2)   The concern here is with these health care providers, not those involved in public health.

The other distinction is between employed and self-employed professionals.   In itself, that distinction is not relevant here.   The concern is with whether the   persons   are   independent   practitioners.   All self-employed   professionals   are   independent   practitioners, but many employed ones are also.   An employed chiropractor is usually independent, that is, has responsibility for diagnosing and treating particular patients or conditions.

The result is a broad concept of healing professions.   Independent healing professionals use specialized knowledge and judgment in treating illnesses and providing for the health of individual clients.   If one wants to use a more restrictive definition of a profession, then one can simply take the argument as applying to all independent practitioners of a healing art or occupation.

The composition of the class of independent health care providers has been changing during the past couple of decades.   Nonphysician independent health care practitioners have increased significantly in both kind and numbers.   Although they have not become widely popular, nurse practitioners are a relatively new group.   More significantly, from 1975 to 1985, the number of clinical social workers increased about 140 percent.(3)

The increase in nonphysician independent practitioners corresponds to a change in the relationships between various health care occupations.   At one time at least, in Britain allied health professions were statutorily defined as supplementary to medicine.(4) So conceived, like a physician's office nurse, they would not often be independent practitioners. But many nurse and lay midwives have their own practices, albeit with physician back-up for emergencies. Consequently, it is better to conceive of the various health professions as having overlapping domains of practice. For example, nurse practitioners, chiropractors, osteopaths, and physicians have overlapping domains with some illnesses and treatments falling in all their domains and some in only one. Likewise, clinical psychotherapeutic social workers, clinical psychologists, and psychiatrists have different but overlapping domains. Whether members of health professions are independent practitioners depends not on their profession's domain but the authority structure in their work situation.

Ethical Aspects of Professional Knowledge

There are at least three broad ethical aspects of professional knowledge. The first aspect pertains to the concept of a professional. Insofar as the term "professional" carries a favorable connotation, its proper application at least relates to value concerns. Professional designation is a sign to the public that the person has special knowledge and expertise on which members of the public can rely. Moreover, certification of a person as a member of a profession confers various benefits. Thus, questions of ethics and justice arise in determining what kind and level of knowledge is necessary for certification.

A second aspect pertains to the allocation of authority and decisionmaking within the professional/client relationship. Who should have ultimate authority to make decisions depends on two factors or "decision maker" principles.(5) The principle of bearing the consequences is that if a person will bear the consequences of a decision, that is a good reason for the person to make it. The principle of expertise is that if a person has relevant special expertise, that is a good reason for the person to make a decision. Neither of these principles is a necessary or sufficient

103

condition for a person making a decision; instead, each points out a major consideration.

Obviously, in the professional/client relationship, any claim professionals have to decisionmaking authority cannot rest on bearing the consequences. Professionals do not bear most of the consequences of their decisions. It is clients whose illnesses persist or are made worse if health care providers make mistakes. Consequently, professionals' claims to authority and decisionmaking must rest on the principle of expertise and their specialized knowledge. However, at least as significantly relevant to treatment decisions, that knowledge can be communicated to clients.

The importance of professional knowledge and expertise then essentially relates to what clients want and can legitimately expect from professionals. There are five kinds of assistance that clients legitimately expect from professionals. First, they expect a diagnosis of their problem. Is the pain in the breast a sign of cancer or just a sore muscle? Second, depending on the diagnosis, they expect presentation of alternative approaches to treating the problem. Third, they expect information about the nature and consequences of the alternatives. Fourth, most people expect and want health care providers to recommend an alternative and provide reasons for the recommendation. Fifth, people often need the professional to carry out the alternative chosen. Whether the alternative involves chiropractic manipulation, psychotherapy, or drugs, the client is usually unable to carry out the alternative alone. Of course, if the preferred alternative is simply rest or exercise, the client does not need assistance in carrying out the plan. All of these steps require professionals to use their special expertise. So even if professional expertise does not justify professionals having ultimate authority over decisionmaking, its use is essential for clients to exercise their authority reasonably.

In connection with these five uses of professional knowledge, the ethical requirement of informed consent is central. To treat patients ethically, health professionals must first have their informed consent.

This requirement particularly pertains to steps two and three -- presentation of alternatives and of information about their nature and consequences. A professional who fails to disclose a reasonable alternative, or a risk or benefit of an alternative, acts unethically.

The third general ethical aspect of professional knowledge concerns the limits of a professional's competence or knowledge. This aspect relates closely to that in the professional/client relationship and could be included within it. However, it is worth singling out for special attention, because it is a judgment that the professional must make. In particular, when should a professional seek a consultation or refer the client to another specialist? The need for consultation arises when a professional is unable to diagnose or determine a preferable treatment for a particular client although the matter appears to fall within the professional's domain of expertise. Most ethical codes require professionals to seek consultations or comply with clients' requests for them.(6) The issue of referral to a specialist or other type of health professional differs, for it concerns whether the problem falls within a professional's domain of expertise. Of course, the two issues are not completely separate, for a professional might consult a member of another health profession or specialty to help make a diagnosis or recommendation for a problem primarily in the first professional's domain. Health problems do not come neatly packaged to conform to domains of professional expertise.

Both consultation and referral relate to a client's concern to have a competent professional. If a problem falls outside a professional's domain of expertise, then that professional is not competent to handle it. If it falls within that domain but the professional lacks knowledge to make a diagnosis or recommendation, the professional does not lack general competence. However, the professional lacks the knowledge necessary to satisfy the client's expectation of expertise or knowledge about the client's particular problem. In either case, the client cannot obtain the expertise sought.

Types and Levels of Knowledge

Before considering ethical issues of limited knowledge, different kinds of knowledge need to be distinguished. Consider the following nonmedical example. The computer word processing package that I used to write this paper contains a program named Word Frequency. I know that it counts the number of words used in a file, the number of unique words, and the number of times each is used. However, I have never used it. Although I have a general idea how to run the program insofar as it is like others, I do not know the specific steps needed to run it. Moreover, because I have extremely limited knowledge of computer programming and have never looked at the Word Frequency program, I have not the faintest idea why or how it works.

This simple example illustrates three different types of knowledge -- knowing how, knowing that, and knowing why.(7) Usually and fundamentally, knowing how to do something is to be able to do it reasonably well. I know generally how to run the Word Frequency program, and by consulting the documentation could probably succeed -- eventually. It would not, however, be appropriate to say without qualification that I know how to run it. As knowing how primarily refers to proficiency at some task and tasks can be done better or worse, there are degrees of knowing how. Some people know how to type or swim or operate computers better than others do. Similarly, in health care, one may to different degrees know how to set a broken leg, conduct psychotherapy of one form or another, perform acupuncture, or provide various chiropractic treatments. Because professionals apply knowledge to practical problems, a considerable amount of professional knowledge is knowing how to do various tasks.

Second, I know that the Word Frequency program counts the number of unique words in a file. Knowing that is knowing the truth of a proposition.(8) I know that the proposition "Word Frequency counts the number of unique words in a computer file" is true. To know how to do something need not involve the knowledge of any propositions. One can speak of people knowing how to do something and mean that they can describe the steps involved in doing it. However, even this ability might not involve knowing that. The directions for doing something are not usually stated as propositions that might be true or false. Instead, they are stated as imperatives which cannot reasonably be said to be true or false. Think of simple directions for taking blood pressure: Place the cuff snugly around the upper arm; pump the cuff up; while looking at the gage and listening through the stethoscope, slowly release the air to decrease pressure; and so on.(9) Professional knowledge includes much knowing that. One knows that red spots on the body are a symptom of measles; that the heart pumps blood; that condoms help prevent AIDS.

Third, I do not know why the Word Frequency program works. To know why is to have an account for something that is the case. For present purposes, it involves an explanation for some fact or event.(10) I know that the Word Frequency program counts unique words, I do not know why it does. One might say I do not know how it does so. This sense of knowing how, knowing how something works or operates, is different from knowing how to do something. Knowing how to do something is to have a skill; knowing how something works is not a skill.

Unlike knowing how to do something, knowing why is dependent on knowing that. One cannot know why something is the case unless one knows that it is the case. One cannot know why the client's sores disappeared unless one knows that they did. Moreover, to know why is usually to know a set of propositions that relate to the one to be explained. To know why influenza produces a fever involves knowing that certain cells react in a specific way and so forth.

Professional knowledge also involves knowing why. In the health professions, it involves knowing how the human body functions. This knowing how can easily be converted into knowing why. One need only pick some aspect of a process and ask why. For example, one could either ask how the stomach and intestine break down and absorb food or ask why food breaks down and is absorbed in the stomach and

107

intestine. Either question calls for a description of the process.

Whether one is concerned with knowing how, that, or why can depend on the level of description. For example, one might ask whether someone knows how to treat a thrombotic hemorrhoid. At this level of description, the question concerns knowing how to do something. At a more specific level it might involve knowing how, knowing that, and knowing why. One might need to know why a thrombotic hemorrhoid occurs -- by a clot blocking a capillary; that the application of heat or surgical intervention will remove the blockage; and how to apply the heat or do the surgery.

Frequently, in health professions difficulties arise because one or another type of knowledge is lacking. For example, a few years ago I had a sore shoulder and ultrasound treatment was suggested. The person performing the ultrasound did not know how to do it well, and as a result I suffered a slight burn from the application of heat. Neither the prescribing physician nor technician knew that ultrasound would work -- it did not. One reason they did not know that it would work (other than the falsity of the proposition) was because they did not know why the shoulder was sore. (This illustration partially explains my aversion to health professionals.)

Knowledge and Treatment

These three types of knowledge pertain in different ways or to different ethical issues. Each type of knowledge can be considered as relevant to some treatment. To begin, consider the ethical import of knowing how to do a treatment. Certification of professionals warrants to potential clients that the professionals know how to treat various illnesses. Yet, certification often depends heavily on pencil and paper tests which primarily ascertain knowing that and knowing why. Although health professions usually require clinical training or practice, that might not be sufficiently emphasized in certifying professionals. Presumably, training programs involve learning how and successful completion of such a program indicates sufficient knowledge of how to do treatments, yet this might not always be the case.(11)

If a professional does not know how to do a treatment, then the client should be referred to another professional who does. The treatment does not fall within the first professional's domain of expertise, and he or she cannot effectively help the client carry out the treatment. Because of the overlapping domains of various professionals, the treatment might fall on the border of one professional's domain but that person not be as skilled at it as another professional might. In this case, the professional ought at least to apprise the client of his or her limited knowledge or skill. If professionals hold themselves out as capable of performing services, then they ought to know how to provide them reasonably well. As knowing how is a matter of degree, there will be difficult borderline cases. Any doubts as to abilities should be resolved in favor of conveying information of possible limitations to clients. Clients bear the consequences of inadequate expertise and have few if any other means of discovering in advance a professional's limited knowledge.

Knowing how to perform treatments can also affect professionals' recommendations of them. Professionals are understandably inclined to recommend treatments which they best know how to perform. It is widely recognized that for angina surgeons are inclined to recommend surgery and internists medical management. The same general point applies in less obvious ways. For example, Dr. Amy's brother Ben, who lives in another city, phones to ask about an operation he is to have on his arm.(12) The physicians planning to do the surgery propose to put a pin in it, and Ben wants to know whether that is the preferred alternative. Dr. Amy then phones various specialists in her town and is told that they do not use a pin. She then phones specialists where Ben lives and is told that the pin method is preferable.

At first impression, one might say that neither group of physicians knows that its preferred method produces better results. In short, there is no professional knowledge here to support recommending one method over another. However, on further reflection, one might come to another conclusion. The physicians in Ben's city know how to do the procedure with the pin better than the procedure without it. Consequently, they obtain better results with it than with the alternative procedure. In Dr. Amy's town, just the opposite is true. In short, if a health professional knows how to provide one treatment better than another and if that professional is to provide the treatment, then other things being equal the former treatment will be preferable.

All these subtleties are masked by health professionals simply recommending one treatment and claiming that it is the treatment of choice. Sometimes a client might have a good reason to prefer one treatment over another and even to change health care providers to obtain the preferred treatment. The situation can be even more important to the client if, for example, it involves going to one type of professional rather than another, say, a surgeon rather than a chiropractor or vice versa.

As the preceding illustrates, knowing how to perform a treatment can be closely related to knowing that it works. A poorly administered treatment is less likely to work than one that is well performed. This point is especially relevant to the knowing that which is necessary to obtain informed consent. A client should be informed of alternative treatments and of their nature and consequences. Because the success or benefits of alternative treatments can depend on a professional's degree of skill in providing each, insofar as possible, the information should be relativized to the professional. A mere statement that "I have had good success with this" is not sufficient ethically, whatever its status legally. To make an informed choice among alternatives, a client needs more comparative information, which might well include that other professionals have just as much success with an alternative treatment.

Because health professionals, especially many of the newer independent professionals, have limited domains of expertise that overlap those of other professionals, the issue professional knowledge and disclosure of alternatives is important. To what extent, if any, are professionals obligated to be aware of and disclose alternative treatments available from other health care providers? The example of surgical versus medical treatment of angina is an example. Should a surgeon note that medical management is available and that internists are as successful with it as surgeons are? A similar point applies to psychotherapy. Some problems that psychotherapists treat, say, depression, are also amenable to other forms of treatment, say, drug therapy. Some psychotherapists may not be licensed to prescribe drugs. Should they advise clients that effective, perhaps more effective, drug treatments are available from other health professionals?

There are three possible claims that might be made at this point. (1) Health professionals need not present alternatives available from other types of professionals even if they know of them. (2) If they know of alternatives available from other types of professionals, then health professionals ought to present them to clients. (3) Not only should health professionals present alternatives available from other types of professionals, but they have an obligation to know of these alternatives.

It is tempting but fallacious to argue for (1) on the ground that clients want the type of treatment available from the professional's specialty, because they sought out that type of professional in the first place. This attributes more knowledge about alternative treatments than many clients have. Moreover, even if one generally prefers, say, chiropractic or psychotherapeutic treatments to others, it does not follow that one does so in all cases. Indeed, it is more likely that clients assume that health professionals will refer them to others when more effective or otherwise preferable treatments are available from other professionals.

One might, however, reject (3) in favor of (2) on the ground that keeping up with other professions places another burden on already overburdened health professionals. By (3), not only should health professionals keep up with their fields, they must also know what treatments are available in other health disciplines. This places an unrealistic demand on them, requiring them to know other professions. One can only reasonably ask that they know their own profession, and that is all that they claim to know. If they do know of treatments available from other fields, then it is part of their fiduciary duty to clients to so apprise them, but they are not at fault if they do not know of them. However, the effect of accepting (2) is the same as that of accepting (1). It throws the burden of knowing which profession can best treat a problem on the client. Often, this presupposes knowing exactly what the problem is, but that is one of the reasons clients consult professionals.

Position (3) is the better one. First, it better accords with clients' limited knowledge. It does not assume that for all problems a client prefers treatment of the type offered by the professional consulted, nor does it assume a client knows the exact nature of the problem before seeing the professional. Second, it is plausibly required by informed consent. Consent is not informed if it is based on only some of the alternatives. One does not make an informed decision to purchase an automobile if one does not know that the dealer across the street offers a comparable automobile for a thousand dollars less. In shopping for automobiles, the burden to discover alternatives can be placed on consumers because they are easily capable of discovering them on their own. As health professions have special expertise not widely available, clients cannot easily discover alternatives.

Third, the burden on professionals need not be overwhelming. They need not know everything about all other health professions; they need only know about treatments available for illnesses and problems that fall within their domain of expertise. Indeed, a psychotherapist who treats depression should, it seems, keep up with the general literature about depression. Moreover, the professional need not know how to do the alternative treatments or why they work, only that they are available and effective. Consequently, the burden does not appear overwhelming. The duty to know of alternative treatments by other professions has been recognized in at least one ethical code.(13)

Knowing why is central to diagnosis. Usually, diagnosis involves going from certain symptoms to the underling cause. To do this, one must know why or how certain conditions (symptoms) are caused. Without adequate diagnosis, professionals cannot present alternative treatments or recommend one, because they do not know what needs to be changed. In short, they do not know what they are treating. A treatment can mask a symptom, prevent accurate diagnosis, and permit the disease or condition to worsen. Consequently, any significant doubts about a diagnosis should be communicated to a client. Obviously, doubts about a diagnosis are a matter of degree and their significance also varies with the seriousness of the problem diagnosed or the alternative diagnoses. Questionable cases should be resolved in favor of informing the client, for the same reasons one should resolve doubts in favor of informing clients of questionable knowledge of how to do a treatment. The client might well wish to ask for a consult even if the health professional does not think the possibility of error justifies it.

Knowing why a treatment works is not essential to its ethical use provided one knows that it does. For example, so far as I know, no one knows for sure why acupuncture works. The traditional account of acupuncture appears quite metaphysical. Nevertheless, like the old man and baptism, one can believe in it because one has seen it done. However, one must know that it works for the diagnosed problem. One needs to know its risks and benefits.

One problem in some of the newer and less prominent healing professions is that practitioners will try their techniques on most anything. There is no objection to trying a treatment on a new problem; indeed, that is how knowledge in the healing professions increases. Sometimes one has a rough theory about how or why a treatment might work for an illness or problem for which it has not been tried, and other times one is just trying anything because all the usual treatments failed. In either case, it is experimental therapy, and the informed consent of the

113

client (subject) should be obtained. For a client to be informed, he or she should be told that the treatment is experimental. Once the treatment proves out, if it does, then one can simply recommend and use it even if one does not know why it works.

It is, of course, preferable to know why a treatment works. One can sometimes improve on it or understand why it fails when it does. Moreover, if one does not know why or how a treatment works, one cannot be as confident that it will not have unexpected deleterious side-effects. Nevertheless, straightforward empirical correlations have been the basis for many effective and safe folk remedies.

Conclusions

Knowledge in the healing professions is ethically relevant to determining the proper domains of different professions, to permitting clients to give informed consent and to make reasonable decisions, and to determining when consultation and referral are appropriate.

Professional knowledge consists of three types -- knowing how, knowing that, and knowing why. Knowing how to perform a procedure is as important for certification of professionals as knowing that or why treatments work. If a professional does not know how to perform an appropriate treatment, then a client should be referred to another professional who does.

Knowing that a treatment has certain benefits and risks, and what precisely the chances of each are, is crucial information. Unless that information is conveyed to a client, informed consent cannot be obtained. Knowing that a treatment has a certain probability of success is often relative to the professional. The better a professional knows how to perform a treatment, the more skilled the professional is at it, the more likely it is that the treatment will work. However, professionals often fail to convey that information to clients, simply claiming that one type of treatment is preferable to another. Health professions have a limited domain, and within their domains of expertise professionals should be aware of effective treatments available from other health professions.

Finally, knowing why is central to diagnosis. Unless a professional knows why a client presents with certain symptoms and problems, he or she cannot exercise any expertise in suggesting alternative treatments and recommending one. However, knowing why a treatment works is not crucial to its ethical use provided one knows that it does. Unfortunately, many treatments in current use have never been reasonably tested for efficacy. It is an ethical responsibility of health professions to conduct research to establish that their treatments do or do not work, or better, what the risks and probable benefits are compared to alternatives.

NOTES

1. See Michael D. Bayles, *Professional Ethics* (Belmont, Cal.: Wadsworth Publishing Co., 1981), pp. 7-8; Eliot Freidson, *Professional Powers* (Chicago: University of Chicago Press, 1986), p. 59. See also Paul F. Camenisch, *Grounding Professional Ethics in a Pluralistic Society* (New York: Haven Publications, 1983), pp. 24-34; Alan H. Goldman, *The Moral Foundations of Professional Ethics* (Totowa, N.J.: Rowman and Littlefield, 1980), p. 32; and Kenneth Kipnis, *Legal Ethics* (Englewood Cliffs, N.J.: Prentice-Hall, 1986), pp. 8-9.
2. See National Federation of Societies for Clinical Social Work, "Code of Ethics," II, in *Codes of Professional Responsibility,* ed. Rena A. Gorlin (Washington, D.C.: Bureau of National Affairs, 1986), p. 173; American Chiropractic Association, "Code of Ethics," Fundamental Principle 1 (1971), in *Professional Ethics and Insignia,* ed. Jane Clapp (Metuchen, N.J.: The Scarecrow Press, 1974), p. 158.
3. Frederic G. Reamer, "Social Work: Calling or Career?" *Hastings Center Report Special Supplement 17* (February 1987): 14.
4. Terence J. Johnson, *Professions and Power* (London: Macmillan, 1972), p. 58.
5. Michael D. Bayles, *Reproductive Ethics* (Englewood Cliffs, N.J.: Prentice-Hall, 1984), p. 79.
6. American Medical Association, "Principles of Medical Ethics," V, in *Codes of Professional Responsibility,* ed. Gorlin, op. cit., p. 101; National Federation of Societies for Clinical Social Work, "Code of Ethics," I(d); American Chiropractic Association, "Code of Ethics," Part I, Art. 1, sec. 7.
7. Cf. Gilbert Ryle, *The Concept of Mind* (New York: Barnes & Noble, 1949), pp. 27-32.
8. This includes any statements that one is willing to say can be known. Thus, on some views, it can include knowing moral claims, e.g., that one ought to keep promises.

9. These imperatives can be defended by hypothetical claims of the form "If one wants to take blood pressure, then one should do such and such." These statements can be true or false. It seems doubtful that one needs to know the underlying hypotheticals to know the specific steps in the process. In any case, one can know how to do something without being able to state or know the steps in doing it. Many good scientists cannot describe the steps in good scientific procedure.

10. Knowing why might be subdivided into at least explanation and justification. Depending on one's view of whether normative statements are capable of being true and false, one might divide justification into logical and moral. For example, that the sum of the interior angles of a triangle is equal to two right angles is logically justified by a geometric proof, whereas the claim that one ought to keep promises is morally justified.

11. I remember a physician who submitted a proposal for the experimental use of acupuncture to an institutional review board and whose training in acupuncture consisted of a three day program.

12. This example is modified from what a physician once recounted as happening to him.

13. See National Federation of Societies for Clinical Social Work, "Code of Ethics," III(b).

TAKING CHARGE OF ONE'S LIFE
Reply to Bayles

By Christopher P. Mooney
Nassau Community College

First, I want to thank Professor Bayles for his paper and state that there are a number of well taken points in it with which I agree, but before I go any further I feel I ought to explain why our featured speaker has a commentator at all. It is not generally the practice at philosophy conferences to include a commentator on the keynote address. I think this is largely a matter of courtesy to the audience, since you ought to be spared controversy at least while digesting your food. Yet the LIPS executive committee felt that an exception might be in order at the Conference since it is common practice to seek a second opinion when deciding upon medical treatment. Ultimately, of course, the choice will be yours as to what you accept and what you reject from both Professor Bayles' paper and my brief remarks.

Before proceeding I would also like to indicate my personal acquaintance with the various healing arts which are the focus of today's conference. Being very fortunate in my health, I have had little need to use any sort of medical expertise (traditional or non-traditional). Also, I seldom use any form of medication or drug since I have found that most of my aches and pains pass quickly. Yet I have long been friends with people who have practiced a variety of the different healing arts being discussed here (and a good number that are not represented). In addition, I have received chiropractic treatment on one occasion to my immediate and great satisfaction.

My greatest practical experience with and knowledge about non-traditional methods of diagnosis and healing comes from acquaintance with an eminent homeopath, Dr. Christopher Cursio, who made remarkable diagnoses via iridology. He treated a good number of people with strict dietary methods quite successfully, but his main complaint about his patients was that they come to him very late in their illness, and they followed is instructions rather sporadically.

In fact, he would stress that the problem facing all members of the healing professions was more a matter of teaching wholesome life styles and encouraging disciplined behavior to the patients rather than curing advanced conditions.

It is obvious that any discussion of the rights and responsibilities of healing professionals must necessarily involve certain assumptions about the rights and responsibilities of patients. I suppose that it all comes down to what we consider the nature and role of informed consent in treatment and what burden of responsibility we place upon the person who seeks treatment Where do we place the burden or the blame when evaluating the patients' right to know and the professionals' right to practice? As Professor Bayles points out, any treatment associated with the healing arts involves both a valuable good -- namely health -- in the hands of the practitioner as well as the mastery of some special knowledge or skill. Thus we are faced with the task of maximizing autonomy for the professional while insuring the highest degree of quality control over the good pursued and the knowledge being used.

As we all know, from the Hippocratic Oath of the Fifth Century B.C. to the American Medical Association's *Principles of Medical Ethics* (1986), healing professionals have attempted to establish clear guidelines to govern their members' behavior and profession. Whatever we may feel about the success or sincerity of these efforts, the simple fact remains that there have always been health professionals who did not qualify for membership within the dominant guild. The Hippocratic Oath contains a prohibition against sharing the special knowledge and skills employed outside the brotherhood in order to protect their purity.(1) And as Mort Sahl once observed, the A.M.A is an equally professional group, for it opposes faith healers, quacks, chiropractors and any other cure that's rapid!

Of course, the problems that arise when there is a recognized and powerful professional group who have control over what is legitimated as appropriate medical treatment and theory and who seek to protect the public from the so-called threat of illegitimate methods are well known. These problems are equally acute in democratic and pluralistic societies, for even in the evaluation of scientific advances and achievements, there is a constant threat that we will pay excessive homage to authoritarian hierarchies and institutions at the expense of individual liberty. It is noteworthy that many of those who would criticize any form of paternalism by traditional, mainstream healing professionals often become extremely paternalistic when it comes to protecting the public against those who would offer alternative healing methods. In this self-styled "New Age" this will not do as a matter of public policy. For despite what we may personally think about the innumerable fads and fancies in the supermarket of New Age followers, individuals must be allowed the right to exercise choice in this area of fundamental importance, namely, one's health care. Moreover, the persistence of the public in seeking out such treatments has recently forced some rethinking about what should be considered legitimate and what should be opposed as dangerous in health care. And I hasten to add that those who believe that the public's support of alternate methods is due only to of widespread fraud and deception on the part of acupuncturists, homeopaths, chiropractors, etc., might well remember that modern American medicine is so filled with exaggerated claims and painless cures that perhaps disappointment with the kind (not to mention the quality) of treatment generally received in physicians' offices, hospitals, and other medical institutions has contributed much to the crisis in current medicine.

The example Professor Bayles gives about different groups of specialists preferring distinct methods of treatment offers a simple example of how every professional group is insular and tends to promote what it knows best.(2) (In philosophy, in fact, this phenomenon is perhaps even more pronounced, as anyone who has listened to a follower of linguistic analysis or a believer in phenomenology knows.) But when we find differing points of view that are not based on some superficial difference of expertise or technical approach, but rather grounded in fundamentally different perspectives and assumptions, the problem is transformed. To use Stephen Pepper's famous terms: we often find ourselves confronted with totally different "world hypotheses"-- radically different "root metaphors" -- that make comparative evaluations almost impossible. After all, if we are to compare things rationally, we must know at lest two of them well. Today, unfortunately, most health professionals seem to have difficulty in keeping pace with advances and techniques of even one approach in the theory and treatment of any given disease or illness.(3)

I know that it will not please some to argue that oftentimes it seems impossible to give an adequate presentation of all the risks, costs, and complications that would be entailed when deciding between two utterly distinct types of treatment-- say, herbal homeopathy and chemical pharmacology. Aside from any other problems, there simply is not enough statistical evidence to guide us in making even the most rudimentary sort of comparison between the two approaches. And, to be sure, supporters of each approach would raise very different issues which they consider should be addressed and/or measured in such studies. The reasons for going to a homeopath rather than a pharmacist are so varied and involve so many other considerations that merely contrasting the treatments and even their "success" rates would be practically futile. It is really a matter of comparing apples and oranges.

To use a religious analogy, I can see nothing wrong with a believer of a certain persuasion urging a seeker to follow that religious tradition without telling him or her to examine every other possible faith or give an analysis of the differences between, say, Christians and Buddhists. Someone might say, "Well, that's different. In religion you're not talking about saving people's lives but just their souls." Perhaps, because we are convinced that the body is really the important thing, we don't worry so much about false doctrines and faiths and think they are protected by freedom of belief, while in health care there have to be other standards and protections since such matters are scientific. Unfortunately, the issue often boils down to the question of whether one

121

accepts the scientific method as the best criterion for determining one's choices. While it may seem obvious to the majority that science should prevail in such areas, it is certainly not the minority view, and it begs the question if one tries to discredit non-traditional forms of healing by saying that they are not validated by scientific theories or methods.(4)

My position comes down to the belief in the responsibility of the individual to inquire independently into the various options. I can no more expect a chiropractor to recommend an osteopath than a Ford dealer to tell me to buy a Chrysler or a Catholic priest to urge me to read the *Dhammapada*. To be sure, these things do happen. Indeed, we probably all know priests who study Zen. (And I recently met a successful Cadillac dealer who told me that he always drove a Mercedes. I remarked, "You can afford to while your customers have to stick with cheaper models.") Expecting non-traditional health professionals to inform their patients about alternate methods of treatment with which they fundamentally disagree seems unreasonable, if not asking the impossible.

This is not the place to go into the analysis of modern medical treatments and their underlying assumptions about the body as a machine *a la* Ivan Illich's *Medical Nemesis*. It is worth noting, nevertheless, that even within the established circles of medicine, there is a greater and greater awareness of and concern about the positivistic metaphysics that lies behind Western medicine. Unfortunately, Professor Bayles does not seem to recognize this, nor does he gives any real indication of seeing the implications of this fact. To recommend that health professionals should explain the alternatives available from other practitioners is not only too optimistic but also too paternalistic from my perspective. While there may be some cross-breeding between certain treatments, e.g., psychotherapy and drug therapy, there is often no such interbreeding between the alternative healing professionals and mainstream medical practitioners.(5)

Ethics does not demand that we exhaustively compare *every* option but rather compare only those options which we judge just and feasible. Of course, this means we will overlook certain possibilities simply because they do not *prima facie* abide by the parameters of our criteria of acceptability. Those who consider the methods of Western science as epitomizing the acceptable criteria for methods of treatment clearly will view certain therapies as nonorthodox. But we must remember that science can only disconfirm our hypotheses, and so much of the rationale in favor of, say, psychoanalysis applies equally to many forms of non-traditional healing. Freud was lucky that he got his M.D. before he developed his therapy. And it was probably smart for American analysts to insist upon medical training as a precondition to admission into the guild of psychoanalysts, even though Freud thought it was unnecessary, if not irrelevant. At least it made them part of the establishment.

Anyone who knows anything about the enmity that osteopaths and the A.M.A in general have exhibited toward chiropractors will hardly hope that the cooperation between these two health professional groups such as Professor Bayles recommends is either practical or likely. We should face the simple situation squarely. If alternative methods of diagnosis, treatment and care are to flourish, we cannot impose upon them the kinds of regulation that have been already developed by traditional medical professionals. Of course, there are those who will say that the potential dangers improper treatments may yield require licensing, regulation and general supervision of all forms of healing and health care -- whether they are traditional or otherwise. Without developing my skeptical, libertarian position fully, I cannot agree with such an assessment, for the same reasons that I cannot see the role of government or quasi-governmental authorities in evaluating political or religious organizations other than when they engage in fraud or tax law violation. I will be the first to admit, on the other hand, that in the case of certain health practitioners fraud may be a very difficult matter to prove. If "Bayer works wonders," however, then crystals may work miracles. It seems that the ideal of statistical and other comparative information *vis-a-*

vis traditional and non-traditional methods of treatment which Professor Bayles would like to see is just not going to happen in the foreseeable future. And the suppression of alternative forms of healing will not work any better than other governmental attempts to control by fiat what the public demands in droves. Thus we must be much more pluralistic than those who so often praise democratic values but become intolerant when it goes against their presuppositions and preferences.(6)

Finally, let me close by saying that whatever form of treatment an individual chooses, it is incumbent upon the patient, except in the most critical situations, to investigate thoroughly the potential risks, costs, and time period that the method of treatment requires. After all is said and done, whatever expertise a healing practitioner possesses, we must assume that he or she is convinced of the value of his or her chosen profession. To expect a non-traditional professional to encourage a patient to seek traditional treatment is just as foolish as to expect a traditionalist to view the New Age with anything but skepticism, even outright hostility. Thus it is the patient which needs to take charge of his or her form of healing, if satisfaction is to be attained. And this conviction, it seems to me, is best protected by an individual's own personal enquiry rather than the self-advertisement of one or another health professional. Healthy skepticism of all healing techniques may be the best way to insure one's health.

NOTES

1. See Ludwig Edelstein, *The Hippocratic Oath: Text, Translation and Interpretation* (Baltimore: Johns Hopkins Press, 1943) for the authoritative treatment of this original code of medical ethics. It might be remembered that Edelstein's attribution of the Oath to the Pythagoreans does not undermine its long-standing acceptance by the broadest spectrum of the Western medical establishment until very recently.

2. Through innumerable stories of a similar sort could be recounted, a good account of the problems involved in seeking a second opinion about a complicated medical conditions can be found in Thomas Nieman, "The Fifth Opinion," *American Scholar*, Vol. 55, No. 4 (Autumn 1986), pp. 536-42.

3. A recent account of fads that have masqueraded as treatment can be found in William Nolan, "Medical Zealots," *American Scholar*, Vol. 56 No. 1 (Winter 1987), pp. 45-56.

4. For a recent treatment of the philosophical and ethical problems involved in making comparisons and conducting experiments about the effectiveness of non-traditional medicine see Wim J. van der Steen and P. J. Thung, *Faces of Medicine: A Philosophical Study* (Dordrecht: Klumer Academic Publishers, 1988).

5. The exception seems to be acupuncture, but even here there are vast differences in the acceptance of this technique in China and the United States by the medical profession. See, for instance, Leon R. Kass, *Toward a More Natural Science* (New York: Free Press, 1985).

6. As this paper goes to press, there is an article in today's *New York Times* (June 30, 1988) about the decision of the journal *Nature* to publish a research report which seemingly confirms the underlying thesis of homeopathy, namely that extreme dilutions of poisons can work chemical reactions. Whatever the ultimate findings of this research, it is not likely to sway a skeptic into accepting homeopathy, and though it may boost

the morale of homeopathic practitioners and patients, I do not see it is appreciably increasing the following. Faith in science is hard to break, and faith in non-traditional medicine is as mysterious as religious experience.

ETHICS AND ALTERNATIVE MEDICINE

By Tziporah Kasachkoff[*]
Borough of Manhattan Community College

The title I gave this paper when I first began working on it was not "Ethics and Alternative Medicine" but rather "Ethics and Non-Traditional Medicine". But the "traditional"/"non-traditional" distinction is both misleading and unhelpful. A few words about why the traditional/non-traditional distinction is not an especially useful one will provide some background for the discussion of this paper.

First, not only does the expression "traditional medicine" not mark off, in any very clear cut way, specific areas on which we might focus our attention, what is regarded as "traditional" is time relative: what is now thought of as "traditional" (like what is now termed "alternative") may very well have a different characterization forty or sixty years from now and what was traditional (as indeed what was "alternative") forty or fifty years ago was -- as we shall see -- different as well.

Second, what we regard as "traditional" is perspective relative. It indicates, at least to some degree, where we stand in terms of our valuation of that form of medicine. What I mean by this is that what we view as "traditional" is generally viewed that way honorifically. Time not only confers "traditional" status on activities and institutions, it "honors" them -- especially when the activities and institutions distinguished by this term characterize something so grand and pervasive as (parts of) our culture or society.

It is worth paying attention to the fact, however, that what has taken place within living memory provides a dramatic illustration of the relatively *short* span of years in which medical conduct and practice may acquire and lose the status of "traditional".

Most Americans who are adults today concede, with nostalgia and some regret, that we have experienced the loss, within our lifetime, of "traditional medical practice". *That* the medical (and nursing) setting has changed over the past forty or fifty years -- for good and for ill -- as well as the ways in which it has changed is not news to any of us. Let me indicate, though only with very broad strokes, which of the many changes we have experienced in our medical encounters are the changes we have in mind when we talk of "the loss of traditional medicine". Up until fairly recently, the relationship in which medical diagnosis and/or treatment took place was, in subtle but still obvious ways, a personal as well as professional one. This is no surprise considering that, until the late 1950s, one generally sought medical advice, diagnosis, or treatment from one and the same physician, one doctor usually attended to all the members of a family, and one and the same doctor served a family over a period of many years. The absence of a high degree of medical specialization meant that a patient saw only one physician for most of his or her medical needs, and the absence of much geographic mobility for both the patient and the doctor meant that the patient saw the family physician for most of his or her adult life. Furthermore, since most health-care needs were met outside the hospital, the relationship between a patient and his or her physician took hold and developed amidst the familiar surroundings of the patient's home and the particular doctor's office, often with the patient's family either present or involved. In this context it was unusual for a physician *not* to know his or her patient's home-life situation, and the social, emotional, and economic factors which affected not only the prospects and probable course of the patient's recovery, but the patient's outlook on his life and illness as well. It almost goes without saying that, clearly, it was the patient -- and in a context that marked him or her as a person -- and not the ailment, which bore the focus of medical attention.

This in brief, and in very general terms, is what we nostalgically remember, or seem to remember, when we lament the loss of "traditional medicine", a lament fueled by our experience of, and disappointment with, at least some aspects of current medical practice.

The most often heard as well as the most poignant complaint of the vast array of complaints that are aired today focuses on the way in which we as patients are depersonalized by our health care system, though some of the forms of this depersonalization have become so commonplace that, already absorbed into new norms of health-care, they are rarely brought into relief even by being noted. (How many of us, for example, will make particular mention of, much less complain about, the fact that practically no health-care services are offered now within the home, and many are to be had only outside a particular doctor's private office?) We have all come to accept that diagnosis and treatment are increasingly carried out with tools that are too expensive, too complex, and too specialized for the resources of physicians in private or solo practice. And so not only do we no longer question the dependence of physicians on the capital equipment and specialized services of hospitals and clinics but, in addition, and probably as a result, we as patients tend more and more to view the hospital or clinic as the locus for what we perceive as the best in modern, technical, medical expertise. This, of course, does not gainsay, nor make more palatable for us, the uniquely depersonalizing features of hospital treatment with which we are all familiar.

We go to the hospital or clinic and, characteristically, we have our medical history taken by one nurse or physician, diagnostic tests given by another, treatment by a third, and if necessary, the administration of drug or physical therapy by a fourth -- unfamiliar procedures administered in unfamiliar settings by strangers with whom there is no history, personal or professional, and with whom, after termination of a particular hospital episode, there may be no further relationship as well. The unfamiliar, the highly technical, even the intimidating have become so expected in the hospital or clinic setting that they no longer seem worthy of particular note. Indeed, within our health-care institutions we are

sometimes satisfied with, even grateful for, mere
civility.

But although the hospital epitomizes the personal
anonymity we have come to view as characteristic of
modern medical attention, our lack, as patients, of
personal distinctiveness is re-enforced in various ways
throughout our health-care system. Both within and
outside the physical institutions of health-care, the
specialization of medical knowledge, of expertise, and
of service have, over the past three decades, eroded
continuity and comprehensiveness of care so that we
often feel differentiated, for greater manageability
within the system, into organs and biological systems
each of which receives attention fragmented along
specialized professional lines. The complaint here is
that organs, not persons, have become the focus of
medical attention and care. Foucault put it well:

> In order to know the truth of the patho-
> logical fact, the doctor must abstract the
> patient.... In relation to what he is suf-
> fering from, the patient is only an external
> fact; the medical reading must take him
> into account only to place him in paren-
> theses.(1)

Of course, we have other complaints as well --
and, needless to say, we also have towards current
medical practice well-justified feelings of deep
appreciation for its benefits and wonders. But my
focus here on those features of current medical
practice which induce our nostalgia for what we think
of as our former medical "tradition", is merely to
direct our attention to the fact that the "tradition"
which sets today's medical practice in such bold relief
as a "predicament" came to an end barely fifty years
after it began.

One has only to read some of the literature
about medical practice at the turn of the last century
and the beginning of this one to realize that barely
two generations ago the medical profession as it
existed in the United States was, for the most part,
regarded *not* with the warm trust and high regard
that we associate with "the traditional medical

practice of our childhood." Rather, there was not infrequent suspicion, distrust, and cynicism. These attitudes were, quite naturally, the result of widespread poor treatments, of misdiagnoses, and often of fraud. Physicians were poorly trained, lacked supervision, and, the public believed, characterized by an avarice unbounded by scruple. (One medical historian has described medical practice of the 19th century as largely irrelevant in the control of disease, except insofar as it was, not infrequently, actually harmful enough to cause the death or damage of the patient. (2)

Were there physicians who were ethical, sincere, well-trained, conscientious, and even -- at least sometimes -- effective? Of course. But the *pervasive* image of the physician as possessed of both awesome technological powers and heroic moral attributes was born only in the early decades of this century. So the odd combination of warmth and reverence which characterizes the so-called "traditional" medical picture existed as a cultural phenomenon for only a brief time in medical history. If we keep this in mind, it will help us to see the current drift towards what is now viewed as alternative medicine in (at least an historically) different light.

What, then, *is* "alternative medicine"? and what moral commentary does its practice in our society constitute?

First off, let me make two observations: Much of what we call "alternative medicine" is not *non-traditional*. Acupuncture and acupressure, for example, have not only been in use for 5000 years, the theory which provides the rationale for their use is the basis for Chinese medicine in general.(3) Chiropractic, i.e., spinal manipulation, was believed to be the remedy for the pathogenic effects of spinal misalignments as early as the ancient Greeks and was fairly widely practiced both then and afterwards. (Hippocrates is credited with having written that one should "look well to the spine, for many diseases have their origin in dislocations of the vertebral column.")(4) Healing through the "laying on of hands", psychic healing, yoga, treatment by means of diet, and especially of herbs, midwifery, osteopathy, homeopathy, and meditation,

131

are all neither new nor recent (though, of course, some are older than others). In fact, almost all of the various modes of diagnosing, treating, and healing which one might refer to as "alternatives" to modern (sometimes called "allopathic"**) medicine predate what we now regard as "established" medical practice and have not been *born* in response to our disenchantment with it.(5) This is not to say, however, that our mounting censure of modern medical practice is not a factor (one among many, I believe) that has made alternative health-care approaches increasingly more attractive to increasing numbers of people.

The second thing to note is that when we speak of "alternative medicine", regardless of the grammar of our talk, i.e., regardless of our grouping of the various non-establishment ways of healing under the single rubric "alternative," we must keep in mind that we are talking about an extremely heterogeneous assortment of ways not only of dealing with but also of thinking about health and illness. "Alternative medicine" covers multiple and varied diagnostic techniques, treatments, theories, therapies, medicines, views, philosophies and ways of measuring outcomes. We must be careful not to generalize too glibly over such divergent practices as homeopathy, acupuncture and acupressure, herb healing, meditation, reflexology, chiropractic, rolfing, biofeedback, osteopathy, and psychic healing, to name but a few.(6)

My caution here regarding generalizations extends as well to thinking that the various non-orthodox modes of healing which are currently being embraced in this country are all undergoing a resurgence in response to a *commonly* perceived difficulty (or set of difficulties) with established medical practice.

To be sure, there *are* similarities in the ways that various "alternatives" differ from conventional medicine (and I shall say something about these similarities below); but the similarities which non-standard approaches to health-care share in the way that they differ from standard medical practice ought not obscure the radical differences among them. Some modes are holistic; some are not; different kinds of problems are characteristically brought to different types of healers; there are different types and different degrees of specialized training involved in the various healing methods; there are different diagnostic techniques, different therapies, different theories of illness and of health(7), and different underlying philosophies.(8) And, of course, within each of the various non-standard approaches there is considerable variation, as there is in conventional medicine, among different practitioners, and among different clients. Responsible talk about "alternative medicine," if it involves generalizations at all, ought to call our attention to the extensive range of practices and practitioners for which these generalizations hold. It ought also to call our attention to something which is subtle but endemic to all health-care choices, and that is the fact that how we choose to take care of ourselves and what we view as doing that, what we regard as health and what we see as its disturbance, endows our health-care choice, whatever it may be, with a social and cultural (some might say "political") meaning that provides a commentary on the way we view ourselves.

Let us turn now to some of the ways in which various non-standard healing modes differ from conventional medicine. (Although, for convenience, I shall continue to refer to these modes as "alternative" medicine, we should keep in mind that this is, in fact, a misnomer. Many of the health-care choices that are referred to as "alternatives" are not embraced as alternatives to established medicine at all but are taken up as supplements or adjuncts to it.)

A list of the ways in which non-conventional modes of healing differ from "scientific medicine" will sound, probably, like a roster of complaints against the medical establishment. Although this is, of course, no accident, there needs to be a great deal more said concerning the *nature* of the connection between the popularity of non-conventional medicine and public disenchantment with the medical establishment. But, aside from merely indicating that health-care choices have to do with more than our disenchantments, I shall not address this issue.

There are several rather striking differences between non-conventional modes of healing on the one hand, and modern medicine on the other. For the purposes of our discussion I shall focus on the following three:

1. Most important, from a theoretical point of view, is the difference in underlying conception of health and illness. Generally speaking, allopathic medicine regards illness as a disordered biological state, determinable and treatable in isolation from social and psychological processes. This is not to deny that modern medicine recognizes, indeed incorporates, a field of study having to do with psychological disorders. But it is to call attention to the fact that when it does this, even here, the illness is isolated from the rest of the person -- the patient is sent to a specialized, and therefore separate, professional whose diagnoses, treatments, and standards of cure are governed by theories and techniques that are not continuous with the rest of medicine. The rest of medicine, meanwhile, working within its own norms of health and cure, remains focused on the patient's biological system and on the biological causes of disease. Little attention is paid to environment either broadly or narrowly conceived. Social, personal, and occupational milieux are, with rare exception, neglected as factors which contribute either to illness or to the appropriate determination of treatment. (9)

To be sure, modern medicine is coming more and more to realize that many diseases (especially those which contribute to chronic incapacitation and death, such as asthma, arteriosclerosis, colitis, heart disease, and hypertension) are diseases whose etiology involves personal, social, and environmental conditions. Despite this, however, modern medicine remains essentially reductivist in its theories of illness and disease, and its approach to cure. Disease is seen -- and some would argue *must* be so seen in order for the "scientific" status of modern medicine to be preserved -- as abnormality, dysfunction or compromise that can always be sufficiently explained in terms appropriate to biology, chemistry and physiology. Reference to conditions that go beyond these categories is regarded as either outside science altogether or, at the least, outside the legitimate purview of *medical* science. As Richard J. Baron -- a physician who laments "the separation of the patient from the disease" -- notes, medical textbooks all too often teach that there is a "pure" disease which is "ideally distinct from any particular patient.... The variations and peculiarities of patients are viewed as 'unfortunate' in that they impede the physician's quest for the disease."(10)

In contrast, non-conventional approaches to health care often assign a pivotal role to the life-context in which the patient's disease or illness is manifest so that environment, beliefs, attitudes, and habits occupy a prominent place in both theories of health and illness and in prescriptions for therapies and cure.

2. As a consequence of their differing conceptions of health and illness, non-orthodox medicine contrasts markedly with "established" medicine in the emphasis it places on prevention relative to cure, the former not only putting the greater weight on prevention, but making it, in fact, the primary focus of health-care attention. Indeed, much of what gets referred to as "alternative medicine" today is considered "alternative" not merely because it substitutes one way of dealing with illness and disease for another, but because it suggests an alternative to the entire notion that to maintain health one must get rid of the deleterious organisms responsible for disease. What is offered instead is the view that certain procedures or regimens conduce to a life of health, and these must be taken up not episodically in response to an incident of illness or an attack of disease, but as life-long habits to promote (if not to ensure) a disease- and illness-free existence. (11)

Of course, not every treatment classified as "alternative medicine" does this. Laetrile therapy, for example, is clearly within the camp of health care which is alternative, non-standard and non-orthodox, but it is also narrowly and exclusively directed only at cure. Nonetheless, prevention is the center of interest of most widespread health-care non-orthodoxies. Health-food and other nutrition-based regimens, to a certain extent chiropractic, yoga and other forms of meditation for health and well-being, rolfing, and even some forms of acupressure, are examples.***

135

3. Related both to the difference in how illness and disease are conceived (1 above), as well as to the difference in emphasis on prevention as opposed to cure (2 above), is the difference in how conventional and non-conventional medicine requires or inhibits the participation of the patient in the health-care process.

Generally speaking, scientific medicine allows and, some would argue, even encourages, passivity on the part of the patient. This is not unacknowledged(12), nor is it surprising -- considering the almost exclusive attention paid to the somatic as a valid basis for judgement and the downplay of the personal and social in both the disease and healing process. I would, however, cite a third factor which, at least to some degree, conduces to the non-participation of the patient: the professionalization of the medical establishment.

Because of the way in which established medicine has developed, popular access to medical knowledge, to medical expertise, and to the tools of medical practice is sufficiently restricted so that responsible self-care is a virtual impossibility. Medical knowledge is to be had only through very costly, lengthy, and intensive schooling; it is accessible only to those who are versed in a highly technical language; and its application is coming more and more to be dependent on the use of highly specialized (and expensive) tools and medicines. It is no wonder, then, that our access to established medical knowledge and techniques must be mediated through professionals in the field. Laypeople are simply not in a position to know the terms of art, nor to use, and in some cases even to understand, the technical tools of medical diagnosis, treatment, and evaluation. As a result, self-diagnosis, self-care, and self-evaluation are effectively ruled out. (13)

Non-conventional health-care approaches, on the other hand, easily engage the active participation of the patient, for the means to such health care are, at least for the most part, readily accessible to the public. Discussion of theory and practice typically appear in the literature without resort to technical or esoteric language with the result that few linguistic barriers bar the way of the non-professional. Furthermore, the modes of preserving health and addressing illness recommended by many non-physician practitioners -- such as proper diet, exercise, and meditation -- are, again, neither technical nor even especially complicated so that no special knowledge or intensive training is required for full participation in, and perhaps even control over, treatment. Moreover, the almost total non-reliance on hospital-based care, and the infrequent use of drugs (and especially of prescription drugs that are available only at high cost) make "non-standard" health-care expertise well within not only the intellectual but also the economic reach of the general public.

There is no doubt that active self-care on the part of the patient finds theoretical support in the underlying philosophies and theories of alternative health-care approaches. But we should not discount as part of what encourages self-care within these systems the simple fact that taking care of oneself is, *within these systems,* an economic and practical possibility.

Some Ethical Considerations Regarding
Alternative Medicine

Let us turn now to some specifically ethical issues regarding alternative medicine. In doing so, we should be careful not to yield too readily to the temptation to judge alternative modes of health care from the perspective of established medicine, a difficult course to follow, since the norms of established medicine are already fairly endemic within our culture. It is difficult, for example, even to ponder the question of, say, how we are to insure the quality of medical care for those who seek diagnosis and treatment outside our established (and regulated) health-care system without using the norms of quality-care suggested by the medical establishment itself. Indeed, even the more general question of how best to promote effective health-care practices is predicated on a notion of what *constitutes* a legitimate health care practice, a notion that in large part derives from the conventional medical scientific ethos. I am not saying here that there is something *wrong*

137

in applying scientific norms as standards to be upheld. My caution is only that we be careful not to use these norms to settle issues which call into question, either directly or indirectly, the norms themselves. For example, if we believe that the State has a duty to safeguard (and perhaps even to promote) the welfare of its citizens, then it is appropriate to ask whether, for the sake of that welfare, the State should paternalistically restrict the access of its citizens to alternative modes of medical treatment. However, we have to be careful not to answer this question using criteria of "welfare" derived from established medical practice but rejected by alternative health-care approaches -- at least not without independent argument supporting such criteria. (14)

The issue I am highlighting here is a general problem that surfaces any time one tries to criticize an institution, practice, perspective, etc., that lies outside the paradigm, when the paradigm has already influenced, and perhaps even determined, the terms and contours of the debate. The trouble here, of course, is that the very questions one wishes to raise, let alone answer, may be compromised by the terms in which they are cast.

The question, then, of the relative merits of alternative versus established medical practice must not be raised without a certain self-consciousness about our use of the notions of health and illness, medical welfare and disease.

With the above as background, let us turn now to explicitly ethical issues. I shall consider three: cost, invasiveness, and respect for personhood.

1. *Cost*: Starkly put, alternative medicine is cheap. We pay less for chiropractic than for orthopedic care (or for the hospital-provided service of a bed with traction devices); we pay less for midwifery than for obstetrical care; we pay less for homeopathic medicine than for prescription drugs; and we pay less for acupuncture and acupressure than for certain neurological treatments and prescription analgesics. Are comparable procedures being compared here? Certainly not. But to ask for comparable procedures is to miss the point. Prevention, for example, is

always, or almost always, cheaper than cure. But there is no doubt that the procedures we use to effect the one are not "comparable" to the procedures used to effect the other. What we are concerned with, then, is not procedure but rather with outcome and therefore what we should be looking at is whether, when we pay more, we are getting better *results* for the money.

The issue here is very difficult to assess since, typically, people go to different health-care practitioners, both conventional and non-conventional, for different *types* of ailments. There are, however, at least some complaints which are brought both to conventional and non-conventional health-care providers and a look at these may tell us something. Obstetricians and midwives, orthopedists and chiropractors, endocrinologists and homeopaths, all see patients who come to one of each respective pair -- at least most times -- for pretty much the same condition. It is to these sorts of pairings that we must look if we are to be fair about how we judge the costs of alternative health-care systems. Unfortunately, though, the kinds of studies that would be useful here are not the sort that generally gets funded -- and so the needed data are scarce. (The one area where there seems to be more than very skimpy and anecdotal evidence is the comparative care offered by chiropractic and conventional orthopedic medicine in the treatment of low-back pain, an affliction suffered at one time or another by, it is estimated, more than twenty per cent of our adult population. Most people who come to chiropractic for treatment of lower back pain have had some previous encounter with conventional medicine *for that particular ailment*, and well over half of these patients come to chiropractic as dissatisfied customers of previous medical attention.) What we need are more detailed data concerning the different types of ailments for which patients seek relief from various health care sources and a comparison of both cost of treatment and success of outcome.

We should, however, bear two things in mind. First, different modes of health care tend to use different criteria for determining whether success has been achieved. Costs may indeed be greater for one than for the other, but not only are benefits, typically, different as well, even what *counts* as a benefit varies from one health care mode to another. Second, the different orientations towards health and disease which characterize established and alternative medicine, the former emphasizing cure and the latter prevention, render comparative studies of the cost/benefit type very difficult to construct. For even given the same outcome and even with the same evaluative stance towards it, the achievement of a given positive outcome by prevention *rather* than by cure may have something more to recommend it than would be apparent by any simple cost/benefit analysis. (15)

2. *Invasiveness*: Another feature of alternative health-care systems which has moral implications for their use is the invasiveness of treatment.

It is by now accepted fact that diagnoses and treatments that are characteristic of the various practices that are called "alternative" are, relative to established medical practice, far less invasive, a fact which reflects well on such practices because of the very high positive correlation between the degree of invasiveness of a procedure (diagnostic or therapeutic), and the frequency and degree of iatrogenic illness and disease (i.e., illness and disease caused by medical intervention itself such as infections introduced by medical procedures, untoward side effects of drug treatments, and surgical mistakes). The general non-invasiveness of the modes of assessment and treatment routinely employed by non-traditional approaches, then, counts *for* these approaches because, simply put, patients are neither especially nor often harmed by them.

It is important to note that the harm of which patients are free when they are free of deleterious iatrogenic effects is illness, disease, dysfunction, and disability as defined by *established* medical practice; it is harm *so defined* that is likely to be a result more of conventional medical care than of non-conventional alternatives. What recommends alternative approaches, then, is at the very least and under the most conservative interpretation, the limitedness of their potential for damage.

There are three things I should add here so as not to be misunderstood: First, although I am claiming that alternative medicine is less iatrogenically harmful than conventional medicine and *to that extent* represents a choice which is to be morally preferred, I am not claiming that alternative health-care treatments are neither harmful nor potentially harmful. The argument here is only that relative to conventional medicine, alternative routes to health-care have a statistically better (indeed, much better) record when it comes to *medically induced* injury and disease.

Second, a word should be said here concerning the fact that the invasive/noninvasive distinction may not be as clear as one might think. Surgery is clearly more invasive than massage; gastrointestinal feeding more invasive than food by mouth. But what of mood-altering drugs? hypnosis? biofeedback? Considering the extent to which these modes of treatment intrude on the very nature of the person, it would seem that a notion of "invasiveness" which does not include them may be too superficial to do justice to the *sorts* of harms that may befall one in the health-care context.

3. *Respect for Personhood:* The third feature of alternative medicine which I should like to call attention to is its focus on patients as whole persons rather than as biological or physiological systems in need of medical repairing. To be sure, not all that qualifies as "alternative medicine" is holistic. However, even where alternative approaches are not holistic, the patient rather than the procedure seems the focus of attention. This may have to do, in part, with the belief, accepted by many of the alternative health-care approaches, that healing takes place from within rather than from the administration of some treatment or drug which is extrinsic to the ailing organism. The view here is that each individual is possessed of self-healing powers, powers that are liberated and helped to regain their potency by the variously advocated alternative health-care measures. (It is easy to see, by the way, how such a view is a

natural partner to the encouragement of patient identification of symptoms, to patient participation in the healing process, and finally to self-evaluation. It is also easy to see how this view is a natural antagonist to the intrusive and invasive procedures that have become part of the routine of conventional medical care. We should remember here the contrast between what, even in the normal case, the obstetrician does in the hospital and what the midwife does at home.)

However, whatever its etiology, one thing is clear: the interaction between the patient and the alternative health-care practitioner satisfies our sense, in a way that current interactions between patient and physician do not, of what is morally appropriate between persons of different expertise but like autonomy.

Conclusion

I would like to close these remarks by pointing out that although my concern in this paper has been to indicate some of the moral issues that surround the choice to seek out alternative medicine both for diagnosis and for therapy, and to call attention to some of the features of non-conventional health-care that bear on our moral responses to it, there are larger questions which the very existence of alternative health-care systems raise: questions concerning the values which infuse any health-care system, and questions concerning the continuity of these values with those that underlie other societal institutions. What moral perspectives do we bring to medicine and how do they shape our expectations of it? Finally, what does it reveal about ourselves as persons that we define our health in one way rather than another, and that we seek to heal ourselves in one manner rather than another?

ENDNOTES

*I am indebted to John Kleinig for very valuable discussions concerning the topic of this paper as well as for his criticisms and suggestions regarding the specific points and arguments I put forth here.

**Throughout this paper I shall make reference to those modes of medical diagnosis, treatment and cure that I wish to contrast with various alternative medicines by use of the terms "allopathic," "established," "traditional," "conventional," "scientific," "orthodox," and "standard." It is not my intention to suggest, thereby, that there are no differences among them. I shall, however, not discuss these differences here.

***I wish not to be understood here as suggesting that there is always a sharp demarcation between what constitutes cure on the one hand and prevention on the other; nor that allopathic medicine is not at all concerned with prevention. Both suggestions would belie the facts. I am, however, calling attention to the fact that, generally speaking, there is a dramatic difference between allopathic and non-allopathic medicine in the emphasis each places on prevention as distinguished -- when it *is* distinguishable -- from cure.

1. Foucault, M. *The Birth of the Clinic: An Archeology of Medical Perception,* translated by A. M. Sheridan Smith (New York: Vintage Books, 1975). See also Raymond Duff and August B. Hollingshead, *Sickness and Society* (New York: Harper and Row, 1968).
2. Duffy, J. *The Healers: A History of American Medicine* (Urbana: University of Illinois Press, 1979).
3. See Dianne M. Connelly: *Traditional Acupuncture: The Law of the Five Elements* (Columbia, Md: Centre for Traditional Acupuncture, 1975) and Manfred Porkert, *Theoretical Founda-*

143

tions of Chinese Medicine (Cambridge, Mass.: MIT Press, 1974).

4. *Manipulation and Importance to Good Health.* See also Hippocrates, *On Setting Joints by Leverage.*

5. See *Alternative Medicines: Popular and Policy Perspectives,* ed., J. Warren Salmon (New York and London: Tavistock Publications, 1984). See also *The Encyclopedia of Alternative Medicine and Self-Help,* Malcolm Hulke, ed. (New York: Schocken Books, 1979).

6. For a discussion of the ways in which, generally, different perspectives inform the definition of disease, see Christopher Boorse, "On the Distinction Between Disease and Illness", *Philosophy and Public Affairs,* 5 (1976); Joseph Margolis, "The Concept of Disease", *Journal of Medicine and Philosophy,* 1 (1976); Tristam H. Engelhardt, Jr., "The Disease of Masturbation: Values and the Concept of Disease", *Bulletin of the History of Medicine,* 48 (1974), pp. 234-248.

7. See the relevant entries in *The Encyclopedia of Bioethics,* Warren T. Reich, ed. (New York: MacMillan/Free Press, 1978).

8. For discussion, see Sander Kelman, "Social Organization and the Meaning of Health", *The Journal of Philosophy and Medicine,* Vol. 5, No. 2, June 1980, pp. 133-144.

9. For both a description and critique of this aspect of modern medicine, see Richard J. Baran, "Bridging Clinical Distance: An Empathic Rediscovery of the Known", *Journal of Philosophy and Medicine,* Vol. 6, No. 1, 1986, pp. 5-23.

10. Baran, *op. cit.*, p. 17

11. See R. H. Miles, "Humanistic Medicine and Holistic Health Care", *The Holistic Health Handbook* (Berkeley, Calif.: And/Or Press, 1978); H. A. Otto and J.W. Knight (eds.), *Dimensions in Wholistic Healing* (Chicago: Nelson-Hall, 1979). For a critique of holistic theory, see *Examining Holistic Medicine,* Douglas Stalker and Clark Glymour (eds.) (Buffalo, NY: Prometheus Books, 1985).

12. See Duff, Raymond, and Hollingshead, *Sickness and Society* (New York: Harper and Row, 1968). See also, J. Katz, "Informed Consent in the Therapeutic Relationship", *The Encyclopedia of Bioethics*, Vol. 2, op. cit., pp. 770-78.

13. For an interesting discussion of the professionalization of medicine, see entries under "History of Medical Ethics" in *The Encyclopedia of Bioethics, op. cit.*; See also Eliot Friedson, *Professional Dominance: The Social Structure of Medical Care* (New York: Atherton Press, 1970).

14. Three interesting articles in this connection are: "The Right to Choose An Unproven Method of Treatment", V. Anthony Unan, *Loyola of Los Angeles Law Review*, Vol. 13, 1979, pp. 227-245; "The Decision to Undergo Acupuncture Treatment: an Expansion of the Right of Privacy", Paul Andrew Drummond, *Houston Law Review*, Vol. 18:378, pp. 373-389 and "Laetrile: Should the Dying Patient Decide?", George J. Annas, *Nursing Law & Ethics*, Vol. 1, No. 7, August-September 1980. The first two treat of the issue under discussion in a rather oblique way; the focus of the third is directly on the issue.

15. Relevant to this issue is the recent rise of Health Maintenance Organizations in this country, and their sponsorship by various health insurance agencies. Until 1973 when Congress, in an attempt to control the rise in medical costs, legalized HMO's across the nation, several states, buckling to pressure from the medical establishment, outlawed them. At present, the HMO Act requires firms of 25 or more employees to offer an HMO as a health benefit option if one is available in the area. This has resulted in a rise in the number of people who subscribe to such organizations -- from 3 and a half million in 1972 to 21 million.

IN DEFENSE OF ORTHODOX MEDICINE
Response to Dr. Kasachkoff

By Leon Pearl
Hofstra University

Tziporah Kasachkoff's paper seems to me to be a polemic against what she calls "modern traditional health care" but which I prefer to call "modern orthodox health care." She begins by contrasting it negatively with orthodox medicine before the late 1950's, and subsequently contrasts it negatively with non-orthodox forms of health care procedures.

Despite the provocative and thought-engaging nature of her paper I find myself in disagreement with her position. My talk is divided into two parts. First I make two general observations pertaining to her paper, and subsequently I try to undermine her argument in a close study of the text.

My first observation is that there is a short passage in her paper where, in the midst of her critical remarks, she concedes some value to present day orthodox medicine. She says "of course we have other complaints as well -- and, needless to say, we also have towards current medical practice feelings of deep appreciation for its benefits and wonders."(p. 130) But why this casual aside remark about a matter of such central importance? For one could not properly begin to evaluate those features of modern medicine which Kasachkoff finds so undesirable such as extreme specialization and depersonalization without considering "the benefits and wonders of modern medicine." The fact is that thanks to modern medicine more people live longer and are in better health than ever before in the history of mankind. And if such great benefits involve some undesirable features, perhaps we ought to learn to tolerate them. Moreover Kasachkoff failed to distinguish undesirable features of present day medical practice such as high monetary expense and excessive hospitalization, which may not be due to modern medical practice as such, but is rather due to the poor medical insurance policies of the government and of the private sector.

146

My second observation is that Kasachkoff failed to mention an important fact which deserves to be taken notice of when comparing orthodox and non-orthodox health care systems, namely the gradual absorption of a number of non-orthodox medical practices into the realm of orthodoxy. For instance in the 1950's obstetricians did not generally practice natural childbirth, but at present it is a standard part of their training. What I am suggesting is that a non-orthodox medicine often functions first as a useful adjunct of health care and is then subsequently absorbed into medical orthodoxy. Notice that medical orthodoxy employs a variety of techniques such as the use of drugs, surgery, chemotherapy, and dialysis. There is no reason why useful health procedures such as acupuncture and chiropractic should not ultimately be absorbed within the realm of orthodox medicine. Kasachkoff's failure to take note of the expanding character of orthodox medicine led her to think of these contrasting medical approaches, i.e., the orthodox and non-orthodox as necessarily antagonistic, as shown near the end of her paper when, contrasting the reliance of non-orthodox medicine on the self-healing powers of the human person, she writes:

> "It is also easy to see how this view is a natural antagonist to the intrusive and invasive procedures that have become part of the routine of conventional medical care. We should remember here the contrast between what, even in the normal case, the obstetrician does in the hospital and what the mid-wife does at home."(p. 142)

I venture to say that there is not a medical doctor who does not think of a human as a self-repairing organism and that when he practices intrusive and invasive procedure he is, at best, eliminating obstacles to the curative powers of the human organism. There simply is no antagonism between both forms of medicine.

We presently turn to the text of Dr. Kasachkoff's paper. In the first part of her paper she notes some of the undesirable features of present day

147

orthodox medicine compared to the practice of medicine between the early 1900's and the late 1950's. In this latter period,

> ..."the same doctor served a family over a period of many years. The absence of a high degree of medical specialization meant that a patient saw only one physician for most of his or her medical need..."(p. 128)

Moreover the physician was likely to know the patient's home life situation and the social, emotional and economic factors which might effect his recovery. At that time

> ..."it was the *patient* -- and in a context that marked him or her as a person -- and not the *ailment* which bore the focus of medical attention."(p. 128)

But today patients are depersonalized:

> ..."We often feel differentiated...into organs and biological systems each of which receive attention fragmented along specialized professional lines. The complaint here is that organs, not persons, have become the focus of medical attention and care."(p. 130)

Depersonalization, continues Kasachkoff, occurs when we go to a hospital or clinic:

> ..."We will have our medical history taken by one nurse or physician, diagnostic tests given by another, treatment by a third, and if necessary, the administration of drug or physical therapy by a fourth -- unfamiliar procedures administered in unfamiliar settings by strangers with whom there is no history, personal or professional, and with whom, after termination of a particular hospital episode, there will be no further relationship as well."(p. 129)

A few comments are in order. Kasachkoff exaggerates the absence of specialization in the good old days. There was specialization in the urban centers in the 40's and 50's though admittedly not to the degree as exists at present. But what I find most puzzling is her use of the term "depersonalization," which she is clearly using in a pejorative sense. I simply fail to see the matter in her light. For when I go to a physician because of an angina problem I want the physician to concentrate his attention on my heart and the arterial system which carries blood to the heart. I surely don't want the physician to examine my brain, my urinal tract, nor that he concern himself with my sexual desires or my hope for salvation. I simply want the physician to concentrate on what is *relevant* to the problem which is likely to include lack of exercise, poor diet, smoking and so on. The physician ought not to focus his attention on all matters that pertain to the person for the very simple reason that economy is fundamental for the efficiency of any activity, and medicine is simply no exception to this general rule. Nor am I thereby depersonalized, surely not in the Kantian sense, for while no doubt the physician in treating me is using me as a means for his enrichment, I am not being used merely as a means, for the objective goal of his professional activity, irrespective of his motives, is my health and betterment.

Nor do I understand why in a hospital setting the fact that one party takes down my medical history, another gives me a diagnostic test and a third treats me, that this constitutes a case of depersonalization. Am I depersonalized if in a department store one person sells me a suit, another mends it to fit me, and a third takes my money? I don't expect the salesman to have the skill of the tailor or the tailor the skill of the salesman. Nor do I have any interest in the department crew, nor they in me other than in the context of the transaction. Why should with respect to the issue of depersonalization the context of the hospital differ from that of a department store? Would you not prefer the physician whose special skill is diagnosis to do the diagnosis and the physician whose special skill is surgery to do the surgery? And why should my relations to the diagnostician and the surgeon go beyond the context of the health care situation?

In summary, I find nothing pejorative or dehumanizing in being "depersonalized" in Dr. Kasachkoff's sense by the practitioners of modern medicine. On the contrary given the proliferation of physiological, chemical and technological knowledge relevant to modern medicine I would not have it otherwise.

In the second section of her paper Kasachkoff deals with the differences between modern medical practices and non-orthodox alternatives. She begins by claiming that they differ in their fundamental conceptions of health and illness: "Generally speaking [she writes] allopathic medicine regards illness as a disordered biological state determinable and treatable in isolation from social and psychological processes" (p. 134). She somewhat qualifies this by stating that modern medicine is coming to realize that many diseases such as asthma, colitis and hypertension involve personal, social and environmental conditions. However, she continues, despite this modern medicine is essentially reductivist in its theories.

In contrast, non-conventional approaches to health care assign a pivotal role to the life context in which the patient's disease or illness is manifest so that environment, beliefs, attitudes, and habits occupy a prominent place in both theories of health and illness and in prescriptions for therapies and care.

Kasachkoff's distinction is overdrawn. Belief in environmental and attitudinal causes of certain diseases is widespread in present day medical orthodoxy. For instance tissue damage associated with ulcers and respiratory disorders are attributed to such factors as personality, stress, outlook on life. There is, however, a difference in this matter between present day orthodox and non-orthodox medicines. The former distinguishes functional from organic ailments. For the latter all ailments are functional. But this difference in theory between the two forms of medicine makes little or no difference in practice. The reason for this is that the influence of psychological factors on organic disorders are not suffi-

150

ciently understood so that curative mechanisms could be developed. No doubt non-orthodox medical theoreticians speak of the whole person but they do so employing abstract metaphysical constructs such as "life force," "prena" or "yin and yang." The medical profession rightfully refuses to endorse such speculative ventures. At best such metaphysical positions are underdetermined theories (thanks to their open texture) relative to the clinical successes which appear to logically follow from them.

The second difference, according to Kasachkoff, is that non-orthodox medicine makes prevention the primary focus of health care; whereas, orthodox medicine is primarily concerned with cure. Again Kasachkoff makes too sharp a distinction. Yoga, meditation and herbalism are undoubtedly primarily concerned with a person's maintaining his well being. But surely people go to a chiropractor or to a practitioner of acupuncture because they are ill or in pain. And no doubt these latter non-orthodox practitioners prescribe health maintenance regimens. But then so do orthodox physicians. They prescribe diets, exercise, the elimination of stress, and so on.

Another difference claimed by Kasachkoff is that orthodox medicine encourages the patient to be passive; whereas, alternative medicines encourages the active participation of the patient. She further highlights this point by complaining about the costly lengthy and intensive training in medical schools and in the construction of a highly technical language understood by a few. This whole discussion I find puzzling -- why should one object to the intensive and lengthy training of physicians? As for technical language, Kasachkoff as a philosopher knows that artificially constructed terminology is useful in order to eliminate vagueness and ambiguity and to aim for a degree of precision not available in ordinary language. The latter of course distances medical knowledge from the comprehension of a layman. But then, how, given the dynamic advances of modern medicine can it be otherwise? Despite the latter a caring physician will, as many of them do, discuss the patient's problems with her on the patient's terms. Moreover it is simply not the case, as Kasachkoff claims, that orthodox medicine encourages passivity on the part of the patient -- as mentioned before, physicians prescribe diet, exercise, medication, elimination of harmful habits and thereby require the active participation of the patient in order to achieve health.

Lastly Dr. Kasachkoff compares the two medicines respecting an issue of morality:

> "[We know that there is] a very high positive correlation between the degree of invasiveness of a procedure, diagnostic or therapeutic, and the frequency and degree of iatrogenic illness and disease (i.e. illness and disease caused by medical intervention itself such as infections introduced by medical procedures, untoward side effects of drug treatments and surgical mistakes). The general non-invasiveness of the modes of assessment and treatment routinely employed by non-traditional approaches, then counts *for* these approaches because, simply put, patients are not especially harmed by them."(p.18)

My mother was kept alive for ten years functioning with a good quality of life in her own home thanks to medications. Now occasionally she suffered adverse side effects such as nausea. Would Kasachkoff count my mother's suffering in her comparative statistical study between the merits of orthodox and non-orthodox medicines? My mother-in-law, an eighty year old woman, had kidney failure and was put on dialysis, and thanks to it she lived in what she considered a good situation for two years. She died of renal failure. Would Kasachkoff also count this case in her statistical study?

Moreover Kasachkoff failed to address a common complaint against non-orthodox medicines, namely that often needed medical care is postponed with resulting harmful effects as a result of a non-orthodox practitioner trying to cure a disease for which he lacks the competence to handle.

It is time to proclaim peace between different medical practices. Unfortunately Kasachkoff's paper does not contribute towards that goal.

ETHICAL ISSUES IN PSYCHIATRY TODAY: AN EMPIRICAL INVESTIGATION

By Beverlee Anne Cox
University of Western Ontario

Psychiatric care and treatment in Canada today is a growth industry. The actual number of psychiatric admissions is increasing even though the overall number of individuals hospitalized at only one time in a psychiatric setting has decreased steadily since 1970 when the trend toward de-institutionalization was first implemented by government policy. In spite of this shift of treatment setting that is suggested by the statistics (from inpatient to a community focus), the fact remains that one out of every ten hospital admissions is officially recorded as a patient with a psychiatric disorder (Ableson et al., 1983).

As the ranks of the psychiatric patient population have grown, the health care system designed to assist them has become increasingly more complex. In most psychiatric clinical settings, interdisciplinary teams are now involved in providing patient care. This has meant, in practice, a more complicated system of decision-making surrounding treatment. Additional factors having a bearing on the situation include: certain ambiguities surrounding the various legislative acts governing the provision of care, the policies (or lack of policies) of the treatment facilities, and the growing militancy of the psychiatric patients themselves through the forum of human rights groups. The end result is that many practical questions concerning care and treatment arise on a daily basis in any given psychiatric setting, and this has produced a situation in which ethical issues are inherently present. This is the subject of the research presented in this paper.

At the outset, it must be acknowledged that many of the difficulties concerning psychiatric care and treatment, and particularly decision-making in psychiatric settings, arise from the lack of a unified scientific model within the field. Instead, there is a considerable diversity of models along a theoretical continuum from the extreme approach of Thomas Szasz (1982), who claims that mental illness is a myth and that the real subject matter of psychiatry is deviant behavior, to the traditional Freudian view that mental illness is analogous to physical illness and can therefore be treated using the medical model approach. That is to say, that there are disease processes internal to the individual, leading to the display of aberrant behavior. This traditional interpretation of the medical model has been widely adopted within psychiatry in Canada and many clinical settings are heavily structured around the use of treatment approaches consistent with the model: psychopharmacology, individual psychotherapy, and electroshock therapy. But at the same time, eclecticism between and among the practitioners of other disciplines represented on the health care team is also prevalent so that, mixed in with the predominant medical model paradigm, one might also find behavior therapy, milieu therapy, and various kinds of group therapies being utilized in any given clinical setting (Cox, 1977).

What does all this mean for the practitioners of psychiatric nursing, the discipline that occupies a central role in the provision of care and the coordination of the psychiatric unit's activities? By and large, one central outcome has been a growing awareness of ethical issues which have come to the fore as psychiatric nurses have attempted to balance the conflicting value systems and demands of other practitioners, patients, and family members. Many of these ethical issues are proving very difficult to resolve, and their very presence reflects in the quality of care being provided to patients. One could postulate that the conceptual ambiguity surrounding the nature of psychiatric disorders, and the lack of systematic and unified treatment methods, laid the groundwork for the emergence of these ethical dilemmas. While nurses generally have a clear idea of problem-solving strategies appropriate to a given clinical situation, when ethical issues come to the fore there is often confusion and uncertainty. The situation is further complicated when dealing with a psychiatric patient population who, by definition, are often not competent to be active participants in putting forward their own views. Obviously, it is of central importance to psychiatric nurses to have a clear understanding of the ethical dilemmas arising in clinical settings today.

Within society today, there is increasing interest and concern with ethical issues, arising in large part from the great impact that science and technology have had on the field of medicine. Enormous strides have been made in developing sophisticated procedures such as organ transplants, methods of reproductive engineering, and complex forms of heart surgery. While these procedures repair the ravages of illness and in some cases, allow the extension of human life, their use has also given rise to many perplexing ethical issues which before the "high-tech" era were not considered a problem. But as Davis (1980) points out, every era has a context from which to view these problems: "The ethical concerns of a society relate to the contemporary human drama, and there-fore develop from a grounded position in time and space. Every ear brings different ethical problems to the fore..."

While general medicine has been struggling with the complexities brought about by science and tech-nology, psychiatry has dealt with advances of a different sort. First and foremost, from a biotechno-logical standpoint, the greatest advance has been the advent of psychopharmacology in the 1950's. Few would argue that the introduction of the major tranquilizers in psychiatry has revolutionized psychi-atric care and treatment for the institutionalized population. Although these drugs provide only symp-tomatic relief, rather than the cure that was once hoped for, they do nevertheless allow thousands of patients to leave psychiatric hospitals and resume a somewhat more normal role in society. Unfortunately, there is a price to be paid since it is now well-established that long-term drug therapy will cause predictable, damaging, and irreversible side effects (Klerman and Schechter, 1981).

The ethical implications of this are now clear; providing drugs to control symptoms (and avert long-term hospitalization) is only a short-term gain.

Ultimately, the patient's health will deteriorate as drug usage is prolonged. What norms and values can be applied in resolving such an ethical dilemma? This example illustrates the type of ethical dilemmas that have emerged in the psychiatric field, dilemmas that touch very closely on the nursing role as it is the nurse administering these medications, often to patients who are unlikely to follow a medication regimen without strong and persuasive nursing intervention.

Many other ethical issues and dilemmas within the psychiatric setting are apparent now when examining the nursing role. Of primary concern at this time are questions concerning the voluntary vs. involuntary patient; the general problem of patient competence, specifically in relation to the giving of informed consent; the use of controversial treatment methods such as electroshock therapy and behavior modification; and issues relating to confidentiality. Here again, psychiatric nurses have daily and very close involvement with these matters and are in a position to influence the decision-making process.

Clearly, all clinical decisions and judgments regarding the above issues carry with them ethical implications. How serious and puzzling these issues are was brought to the writer's attention through ongoing discussion with nursing staff on an inpatient psychiatric service in London, Ontario. Through the establishment of a dialogue about some of the problems the nursing staff were experiencing, a decision was reached to investigate, in a systematic manner, all such ethical problems as they arose during a designated period of time.

The research questions to be addressed in this project were: a) are there ethical issues/dilemmas occurring on the unit? b) If so, what are the nursing staff's perception of these issues? c) How can these issues be described? It was the investigator's intention to determine what, in the nursing staff's view, could be described as an ethical issue or dilemma rather than to impose a conceptual framework in which operational definitions of ethically complex situations were supplied.

The purpose of utilizing this approach was to derive empirically the staff's *perceptions*, assuming that this information could provide the basis for using a grounded theory approach in order to construct, eventually, a taxonomy of ethical issues which could then be tested for verification in other psychiatric settings. The grounded theory approach, now well-established in the social sciences, allows the researcher to construct categories, code the qualitative data and shape the data from analytic interpretations, thus leading to the construction of a theory (Glaser and Strauss, 1967). Since the data for this project were to be actual verbal self-reports of critical incidents on the unit, this was not only a logical but necessary approach to the material.

This research project took place on a twenty-bed psychiatric inpatient service which is part of a large teaching and research hospital. Because of its university affiliation, the hospital has staff and students from all disciplines (medicine, nursing, psychology, social work and occupational therapy) operating as a multidisciplinary team on the psychiatric unit. The patients are primarily sent to the unit by referral and can generally be described as acutely ill, many having been hospitalized previously, and representing a wide range of the major psychiatric disorders. Many different kinds of therapeutic modalities are used with these patients: all forms of psychotherapy, including group and family therapy, electroshock therapy, art and occupational therapy, milieu treatment and most importantly, drug therapy. The unit, its staff, patients, and treatment approaches are representative of a typical university psychiatric inpatient service today in Canada. The philosophy of the unit is centered on the provision of individualized and patient-centered care. The staff-patient ratio is considered to be highly satisfactory and contributes markedly to the efficiency of the unit's operation. The average patient stay is approximately four to six weeks.

Since the decision had been made at the outset of this project to utilize an empirically-derived approach, staff members were not given any operational definitions of ethics, ethical issues and/or

158

dilemmas. It was the investigator's intent to capture the staff's undiluted perceptions of these matters. Prior to the actual data collection period of four weeks, meetings were held with the staff in order clearly to set the stage for data collection. At these meetings a set of guidelines concerning data collection was reviewed and the project's methodology was explained: all staff were asked to provide on audio-tape, a report of any incident occurring on the unit that had, for them, an ethical dimension. They were, of course, assured complete confidentiality and anonymity as the data were disguised by giving them code numbers for their reports.

The response during the data collection was highly positive. Ninety percent (90%) of the staff had volunteered to participate (out of a total of eighteen possible participants). Twenty-three self-reports were submitted by eight different staff members. The audiotaped data were transcribed verbatim and these transcripts provided the basis for the first stage of the content analysis.

Initially, the themes and categories were identi-fied and separated into three groups: a) those ethical issues identified by the subjects as such and validated by the researcher as bona fide ethical issues; b) those issues considered to be ethical ones by the staff but not by the researcher; and c) ethical issues that emerged from the data which had *not* been identified by the staff. The following table identifies the significant ethical issues:

ETHICAL ISSUES IDENTIFIED
BY THE STAFF AND/OR IN THE DATA

1. Truth-telling/Information-Giving

2. Patients' Rights

3. Role/Trust Within Health-Care Team

4. Informed Consent

5. Objectionable Means

6.   Confidentiality

7.   Therapeutic Process

8.   Paternalism

9.   Job Responsibility

10. Objectivity/Appropriateness
     of Health Care

Many of these problems identified empirically by the staff are representative of areas that are already reflected in the biomedical ethics literature. In Table I (next page), the frequency and range of the issues, as identified by each respondent, is indicated.

In summary, there were six reports of issues relating to the first category, truth-telling and information-giving. Of those six reports, five were considered to be genuine ethical issues. Patients' rights was reported as a subject area three times, but only once did a report actually involve an ethical matter. Roles and role relationships, focusing on issues surrounding trust within the multidisciplinary team, emerged as a separate category but did not meet the criteria for classification as an ethical issue although staff were expressing genuine concerns. Informed consent became a separate category with four reports submitted, two of which were considered to be ethical issues, and two were representative of other clinical concerns. Questions about the use of objectionable means of treatment arose once. Issues concerning confidentiality were reported seven times, and five of the reports were actual ethical issues, two were not.

The final four categories, therapeutic process, paternalism, job responsibility, and the appropriateness of health care arose a total of seven times, and except for the one report of paternalism, were all considered to be questionable in terms of their ethical validity.

To illustrate the nature of the data, three self-reports are briefly summarized below:

Table I

Code:
a) one star - ethical issues identified by staff and validated by the researcher
b) two stars - those issues considered to be ethical by the staff but
   questionable by the researcher
c) 0 stars - other concerns

ETHICAL ISSUES	A_1	A_2	A_3	A_4	A_5	A_6	C	E	J_1	J_2	J_3	J_4	J_5	J_6	K_1	K_2	K_3	K_4	K_5	N	P	T_1	T_2
Truth-telling/ inform-giving	√*	√*	√*				√*										√*		√**				
Patient's rights	√**														√**	√*						√**	√**
Role/trust within Health Care Team	√**					√**	√*																
Consent		√				√*	√*								√*		√**						
Objectionable means	√*																						
Confidentiality		√			√**						√*	√*		√*				√*		√*			
Therapeutic process				√**	√**																		
Paternalism						√*																	
Role Responsibility							√**						√**										
Objectivity/ Appropriate Health Care										√**													

161

In Situation A, a staff member (nursing) has discovered that a patient who was scheduled for electroshock therapy was told by the physician that the machine was malfunctioning and he would have to be transferred to another hospital to receive the treatment. Since many other patients had been exposed to this machine, the immediate concern was that great anxiety would be created among the patients. Then the nurse, in discussing this incident with the physician, learned that he had only *said* the machine was malfunctioning because he thought this was an appropriate way to convince the hospital administration to buy a more sophisticated machine. The staff member reports that in discussion with colleagues there was general consensus that it was unethical to deceive the patients, create possible anxiety, and in general to attempt to manipulate the administration in this way. The staff member also felt deceived by the physicians.

This incident did raise numerous important ethical issues and is analyzed as follows: a) the primary issue is "truth-telling and information-giving." False information was given to the patient and this information may, or may not, have become common knowledge among the patient group, many of whom had already received electroshock treatments from the "malfunctioning" machine. The second aspect of deception concerns the physician's deception of the staff regarding this matter as he did not acknowledge that the machine was not actually malfunctioning until confronted by a staff member who asked for further information. b) This situation also raises the question of patients' rights. Were any rights violated? Undoubtedly so, since patients have the right to the truth regarding their care and treatment. This may have been, in fact, more of a legal issue than an ethical one, but it also underlines the third category of concern: trust within the health care team since the reporting staff member perceived herself as having been the object of deception on the part of the physician.

A final, but important issue here is classified in the data analysis as "objectionable means." On the one hand, it could be said that the doctor is to be commended for attempting (through subtle coercion, unfortunately) to secure a better machine for his patient; however, are the means by which the doctor attempted to achieve these ends ethically acceptable? From an ethical standpoint, the question must be asked as to whether he had a right to proceed in the way he did *regardless* of the condition of the machine. He was, in fact, using the patient as a political lever and engaging in deception with the staff.

In Situation A, secondary issues in this case involved the expression of legal liability; the staff's need to maintain patient safety at all times and wondering if this had been violated; and the issue of trust between and among all members of the health care team. It is the perception of the reporting staff member that this trust had been violated.

In Situation B it is reported that a patient on the unit (who is psychotic, suicidal and hallucinating) had not been certified by the admitting physician, i.e., she was not on involuntary status. However, he had stated on the chart that if the patient attempted to leave the unit, she should be restrained and then certified. The patient had not been informed of this and the staff member reporting on this expressed grave reservations concerning the ethics of the situation since legally (in Ontario) voluntary patients cannot be restrained from leaving hospital. But more importantly, the staff member felt that the patient was being deceived about the circumstances of her hospitalization.

The major ethical issue identified in this case concerns information-giving. The staff member believed that the doctor should have told the patient that her disturbed behavior would influence her status in hospital and could lead to being certified. The patient is perceived as being in a powerless situation with no control over the outcome. Other subsidiary concerns are also identified: legal responsibility is considered a primary concern since there appears to be some ambiguity regarding the physician's directive. This directive is also in violation of standard hospital policy, also a major concern as reported by the staff member. Finally, there is a question concerning areas of responsibility, and the delegation of responsibility. By what authority has the physician issued the directive to other staff members to restrain the patient? Can this be justified on ethical or policy grounds? And what would the view of the hospital administration be if this situation were scrutinized from a policy standpoint? These questions illustrate the complexity of this case. Unfortunately, this is a situation which is not at all uncommon, one in which the ethical dimensions are often left unexamined.

Situation C concerns a psychiatric patient in hospital who is scheduled to undergo a minor surgical procedure. There was a question, at the time he signed the consent, of the possibility of a second diagnostic procedure being carried out while he was under the anesthesia. It was discovered (by the staff member) prior to his going to surgery that indeed the second procedure was in all likelihood, going to be carried out. The attending surgical resident conveyed this news to the staff member who suggested the resident inform the patient of this himself. Because he was "pressed for time," he declined to do so, thus leaving the nursing staff member to do it.

In the nursing staff member's report here, two ethical issues were identified, the first concerning his view that the patient was not provided with complete information; and secondly, that there had not been a true "informed consent" obtained from the patient

164

because of the lack of clarity about the second procedure. Certainly a case can be made for stating that the information was incomplete: the nature of the procedure and its implications, including risks and benefits, had not been fully explained to the patient.

Other issues in this situation that go somewhat beyond ethical concerns but were nevertheless reported by the staff member are in the category of roles and role responsibilities within the health care team as well as legal concerns. Regarding the former, there is some expressed confusion about just who is responsible for information-sharing and obtaining a fully informed consent, and this confusion is reported as a kind of disagreement between two members of the health care team. Finally, because this is a serious situation, (involving surgery and general anesthesia) some concern is expressed about legal liability, and rightly so.

In Table II (next page), there is a representation of all of the concerns that were expressed by the reporting staff members that were classified in the data analysis as going beyond purely ethical issues or dilemmas, i.e., these were the concerns that most often could be classified as clinical, legal, or having to do with responsibilities, professionalism, and role relationships.

It is noted that legal concerns are pre-eminent here, having been identified in seven reports. Questions of responsibility of the individual reporting, or perceived responsibility of others, was reported five times. All of the other issues appeared in the data, two, three or four times. The total number of additional concerns reported were thirty, all of which added a significant perspective to the data analysis since they represent important clinical matters. These issues, as described in the self-reports, were indicative of the staff's concern for the quality of patient care that was being delivered, and in most instances questions were being raised about the possibly adverse effect these matters might have on the patient's care and treatment.

In summary, five recurrent themes were noted in the data, all of which give some indication of the complexity of the issues involved in psychiatric care

Table II

ADDITIONAL CONCERNS

ETHICAL ISSUES	A1	A2	A3	A4	A5	A6	C	E	J1	J2	J3	J4	J5	J6	K1	K2	K3	K4	K5	N	P	T1	T2
Legal Concerns	✓		✓	✓	✓		✓	✓	✓			✓									✓		
Patient Care	✓		✓													✓	✓						
Role/trust within Health Care Team	✓														✓	✓	✓					✓	✓
Doctor-nurse relationship	✓						✓		✓						✓								
Therapeutic Nature of inform		✓																✓					
Responsibility			✓	✓	✓					✓				✓								✓	
Role of nurse							✓																
Doctor/patient Relationship																							
Professionalism (role of doctor)														✓					✓				
Decision to document inform																		✓					

166

and treatment today. Just as the discipline is without a truly scientific approach to care, so is it also lacking in a consistent approach to the resolution of ethical matters of concern to both patients and professionals alike.

ETHICAL ISSUES IN PSYCHIATRY
Recurrent Themes

I.   Truthtelling/information-giving

II.   Confidentiality

III.   Informed consent

IV.   Trust

V.   Legal concerns

The most predominant and recurrent theme to emerge was that of truth-telling and information-giving. Although in each separate report there were obviously distinct problems to consider (because the facts or circumstances of the cases differ) the staff expressed a predominant concern about telling the patients the truth and giving them appropriate information about their diagnoses, circumstances of hospitalization and proposed treatment plan. Often, but not always, this concern is linked with certain issues concerning consent and personal legal responsibility. A separate but related issue was the expressed concern (and often confusion) about when information should be withheld from the patient on therapeutic grounds.

The second most noted concern was that of confidentiality. Here again, there is widespread concern and confusion regarding what kind of information should be treated as confidential, and under what circumstances confidentiality should be breached. A troubling issue for many staff members was related to when confidentiality might be violated for therapeutic reasons.

The theme of informed consent is raised throughout the data. There are many difficult aspects

167

to this issue; in particular, the staff are concerned that consent procedures might be inadequate, and, in one instance, that the means used to obtain the consent might have been inappropriate.

Another recurrent theme is that of trust between and among members of the health care team and/or with the patient. It is repeatedly asserted in the data that a feeling or sense of trust is absolutely essential to the effective functioning of the health care team; whenever that sense of trust is perceived to have been violated, staff members expressed concern about their ability to provide optimal care. Clearly, there are secondary issues here as well concerning authority, status and perceived role responsibilities toward others.

The final recurrent theme of legal responsibility was noted throughout the data and in most cases, was presented in a personalized manner, i.e., the staff member reporting the concern was questioning whether he/she was assuming some legal liability because of the actions of others. This arose most frequently in regard to compliance with policies, institutional rules and/or current legal codes.

This research project demonstrates the interest among a select group of professionals in moving toward a resolution of their perceived ethical dilemmas. Their willingness to provide the data and to enter into discussion with the researcher was a clear indication of a high degree of interest in ethics and a commitment to providing excellent patient care. Now that many of the ethical issues have been identified, the next step will be to undertake a series of staff discussions using a theoretical framework for the resolution of the ethical issues emerging from this project.

The complexity of these ethical issues identified by the staff are deserving of further study inasmuch as the overall goal of these endeavors is to improve the quality of care for patients on this unit. Considering the difficult problems that psychiatric patients present for staff members in the areas of competence, autonomy, and informed consent, it is clearly in the staff's best interests to have guidelines for ethical behavior formulated in such a way that a consistency of approach may be applied in any given situation. As Szasz (1982) has noted: "Anything that people *do* -- in contrast to things that happen to them -- takes place in a context of values. In this broad sense, no human activity is devoid of ethical implications." While Szasz was referring in this passage to what psychiatrists do, the statement could apply with as much relevance to what nurses do with patients. In considering that nurses are with patients twenty-four hours a day, as opposed to much briefer contact by other professional disciplines (at least in inpatient settings), one could postulate that the number of ethical dilemmas encountered by nurses is far greater.

Of course, it should be noted in closing that focusing only on ethical issues will not, in and of itself, resolve many of the significant problems with the health care system alluded to at the outset of this paper. As Jackson (1985) asserts: "The present health system is in a state of chaos and creative ferment, depending how you look at it." This is even more evident when directly applied to the field of psychiatry. Significant efforts will be required on the part of professionals, public policy makers in the government, and the consumers of health care alike if the serious problems within the system are to be redressed.

REFERENCES

1. Ableson, J., Paddon, P., Strohmenger, C., *Perspectives on Health* (Ottawa: Statistics Canada, 1983), pp. 90-92.

2. Cox, B., *Communication Systems in Psychotherapy* (Simon Fraser University, Burnaby, B.C., Doctoral Dissertation [Unpublished]), 1977.

3. *Davis, A. and Aroskar, M., Ethical Dilemmas and Nursing Practice* (E. Norwalk, Ct: Appleton-Century-Crofts, 1983).

4. Davis, A., and Krueger, J. (eds.), *Patients, Nurses, Ethics* (New York: AJN Publishing Co., 1980), pp. 3-8.

5. Edwards, R. (ed.), *Psychiatry and Ethics* (Buffalo, NY: Prometheus Books, 1982).

6. Glaser, B., and Strauss, A., *The Discovery of Grounded Theory: Strategies of Qualitative Research* (Chicago: Aldine Publishing Co., 1967).

7. Hunt, R., and Arras, J. *Ethical Issues in Modern Medicine,* (Palo Alto: Mayfield Publishing Co., 1977).

8. Jackson, R., "Issues in Preventive Health Care", *Science Council of Canada* (Canada, Ontario, 1985).

9. Jameton, A., *Nursing Practice: The Ethical Issues* (Englewood Cliffs, NJ; Prentice-Hall, 1984).

10. Klerman, G., and Schechter, G. "Ethical Aspects of Drug Treatment," *Psychiatric Ethics*, Bloch, S., and Chodoff, P. (eds.) (New York: Oxford University Press, 1981), pp. 117-130.

11. Szasz, T., "The Myth of Mental Illness," *Psychiatry and Ethics*, Edwards, R., (ed.) (Buffalo, NY: Prometheus Books, 1982), pp. 9-28.

12. Van Hoose, W., and Kottler, J., *Ethical and Legal Issues in Counselling and Psychotherapy* (San Francisco: Jossey-Bass Co., 1982).

13. Williams, J., *Biomedical Ethics in Canada* (Lewiston, N.Y.: The Edwin Mellin Press, 1986).

Note: The author gratefully acknowledges the assistance of Mrs. Jean Rollond, Nursing Manager

(Psychiatry), University Hospital, London, Ont., and her staff in the collection of data for this project.

SOME METHODOLOGICAL ISSUES IN PSYCHIATRIC ETHICS
Rejoinder to Cox

By Salvator Cannavo
Brooklyn College

What I find engaging about Dr. Cox's investigation is that she uses an empirical approach for a project in ethics, an area where the standard method of inquiry has been philosophical. This approach, known mostly to sociologists as grounded theory, is intended as a strategy for categorizing ethical issues. But despite its appeal and freshness of promise, the method, for the purposes of her investigation, does leave me with serious doubts.

My concerns are actually two -- one generally philosophical, the other a matter of methodological refinement. Consider the philosophical one first. It has to do with an old problem that arises when purely factual findings are used to arrive at ethical conclusions. By asking staff members to submit reports of critical incidents which they see as having ethical dimensions, the project takes on the character of a sociological investigation. The social group is the psychiatric staff; the characteristics focussed upon are its ethical perceptions. Up to this point, therefore, the investigation belongs to a *de facto* sociology of ethical concepts and perceptions rather than to ethics proper.

But, Dr. Cox's investigation also takes a turn away from the empirical. She requires that individual reports be reviewed by an expert -- in this case, herself. It is she who validates the ethical content of reported issues before the reports become *bona fide* data. In this way, the investigation, departs somewhat from grounded theory sociology, and moves closer to being a more analytical or, as one might say, philosophical study. The perceptions of staff members are no longer the sole basis for generating concepts. They are processed analytically against a background into which they are incorporated and which then becomes the total basis for the ensuing review, codification and analysis. On such a view of the study, staff reports can be seen as merely suggestive paradigm cases, paradigm cases that could have been readily produced simply as imagined possibilities.

One can, I suppose, still insist on calling the project empirical in the sense of regarding the submitted data as the primary and sole basis of the study. But then, this minimizes, at least, the researcher validations. More ominously, however, the specter of a fact-value confusion begins to emerge, and the results of the investigation threaten to take on a curious twist. Imagine for a moment that we were to extend our project by making ethical evaluations and recommendations for resolving the issues that have been identified and categorized. Would we then say that our recommendations had been fashioned to resolve issues that actually *have* ethical dimensions or, instead, issues that are merely *perceived* by the staff as having ethical dimensions? In other words, would our recommendations count for results in medical ethics or results in applied psychiatric sociology? I am strongly inclined to believe that there is a real difference between these two alternatives. In support of my belief I would want to point out that the matter of which issues are perceived to be ethical by some group, to some extent, depends on which group does the perceiving. But this dependency is not generally thought to hold for issues that are genuinely ethical.

Finally, we would expect our empirical findings to be sufficient for deciding what we are supposed to understand by an ethical issue and perhaps also what we *ought* to recommend for resolving it. Alas, we are brought here to the brink of the old but compelling naturalistic fallacy objection. How can *de jure* conclusions ever be derived solely from purely *de facto* sociological findings? Admittedly, some contemporary philosophical analyses, toward which I have strong philosophical leanings, have played havoc with the fact-value distinction and thus taken some of the bite out of this sort of objection. But one still likes to see how the objection is met in particular contexts.

My second concern has to do with how Dr Cox's categories apply specifically to psychiatry. My doubts this time stem from the kind of empirical data which is used for generating the desired categories. As we know, this data consists of incidental episodes reported by staff members. But, Dr. Cox's expository passages illustrate emphatically how her own background of knowledge can, by itself, that is, without the use of fresh data, point up the uncertainties, hazards, and low yield trade-offs characteristic of psychiatric treatment. The contrast with all other branches of medical service, is deepened when she notes how psychiatry is disunited, even on clinical levels, by theoretical rifts at its very foundations. Thus not only is the researcher in this subject strongly familiar with the relevant features, on-going circumstances and ethical quandaries of our psychiatric services, but she is clearly aware of their differential bearing on our ethical concerns. Indeed, this background also takes account of the present-day literature of medical ethics with its full armamentarium of ethical concepts and distinctions. We have here a total background which by itself, can be superbly indicative of those aspects of psychiatry that have major ethical dimensions. It can be reflected upon and analyzed intensively to yield not only the desired categories but also a network of hypotheses relating them. These, I believe are strong grounds for maintaining that, studying episodal incidents, thought by the members of some group to have ethical dimensions, is not necessary for the purposes of the investigation we are considering. The strategy I would be inclined to favor therefore, *in lieu* of grounded theory, or any other field study or experimental approach, is one which explicates and interrelates concepts and information already in hand. What I am recommending is standard conceptual and critical analysis. (Call it philosophical analysis if you like.) Indeed, as I have already noted, a lucid analysis over terrain that is obviously already familiar is precisely what Dr. Cox gives us at the very beginning of her discussion and elsewhere. How the gathering of anecdotal data from staff-members can possibly advance the major aspects of her study is a matter about which I have much doubt.

But, our empirical approach here is, I believe, not only unnecessary; it is also insufficient and even detrimental. Indeed focussing on incidental episodes can and, I believe, in this case does compromise the pertinence of the emergent categories. The reason for this is that by using dispersed happenstance incidents as data, vaguely thought to be germane to the purposes of an investigation, a study can easily be sidetracked into considerations that have, at best, only a general bearing on these purposes. To illustrate this point we can go directly to our categorizations and take just two as examples. These are *information giving* and *informed consent*. I would like to suggest that these categories are simply too general for their intended domain of application. Indeed, these categories could have readily emerged from a similar investigation in a general hospital. Again, the root of the problem seems to be the incidental nature of the data indicating the category. Recall the episode about informing the patient of the possibility of an additional surgical procedure during anesthesia. This scenario, though perhaps appropriate for an investigation in general medical ethics, has little to do with the very special difficulties that arise in psychiatric contexts. We seem to have here a serious loss of pertinence. I wonder for example, how the resulting general notion of *information-giving*, by itself, can ever yield any of the ethically laden concerns that arise in strictly psychiatric. situations. Here are a few that easily come to mind: Apprising patients of the predictable hazards and low-yield cure rates of psychiatric treatment; presenting patients with the hard fact that there are radically different alternatives for treating and managing psychiatric disorders, with little clinical or theoretical basis for deciding the choice; processing information so that it can be understood by patients with some cognitive impairment; giving potentially injurious information to seriously disturbed patients; informing the family or friends in case a patient has no ability to process information; holding hearings of record for uninformable patients where there are no relatives or friends, and so on. Some of these more specific concerns like that of consent giving under special psychiatric limitations are in fact alluded to briefly here and there in the discussion. But it is not clear whether the researcher's perceptions in these matters spring from the data or from her own background and creative thinking. One might want to grant here that a set of categories specifically narrowed along such special lines could seem too specific for the kind of generality and elegance usually required of any taxonomy. But without the specificity, the desired pertinence is lost except in the most trivially general senses. (Information giving of one sort or another is normally obligatory in all human decision making.)

It is easy to imagine similar refinements for the general concept of *informed consent*. In psychiatric contexts, the circumstances are analogous to those just listed for *information giving*. One might note here that this time the autonomy and overall person-hood of the patient seem to be even more precari-ously at stake, given the cognitive and emotional difficulties which encumber her/him. *Informed consent*, therefore, like *information giving*, could well be supplanted by more specific concepts, tailored to the unique aspects of the psychiatric domain. In the very jargon of grounded theory one might want to express this by saying that what is desirable here is a set of categories that are less formal and more substantive.(1)

Before concluding, I would like to pause briefly for what is perhaps a more tenuous consideration, but one which has an additional bearing on the pertinence of our derived categories. This time, my concern is a more specifically semantical one.

Let me note, to begin with, that there seems to be no way of grasping the full meaning of a concept without relating it to its domain of application. The data matrix which ostensibly first generates the concept is by no means negligible as a part of this domain. In this case, therefore, where the derived categories in themselves betray nothing especially characteristic of psychiatry, one might reasonably want to go back to the original observational context and data for clues about how to implement these categories. (The term 'mass', in quantum mechanics, for example, does not have quite the same meaning as it does in classical mechanics. And this is due not only to formal differences between the theories but also to the kinds of experimental contexts first associated with each theory.) But unfortunately, in the present investigation, the empirical context consists entirely of incidental episodes in which the psychiatric content tends to get lost in the shuffle. For, inevitably the semantical range of the data randomly broadens to the most general medical levels and away from specifically psychiatric ones. As a result our categories, rather than becoming *simply* less specific become referentially more ambiguous and eventually lose touch with the intended domain of application. Often this is O.K. The proper assignment of initial conditions usually provides all the necessary specs. Psychiatric services, however, are so different from virtually all other medical contexts that the assignment, or better -- discovery -- of appropriate initial conditions would itself require a new research project. In effect, therefore, the generality of the categories induced by the free-floating data base of critical episodes amounts to an undesirable shift of emphasis from abnormal to normal ethical contexts. The point here is that this shift of emphasis imparts to the categories an altered sense that contributes heavily to the loss of pertinence about which I mean to caution. Surely, the notion of *information giving* or that of *informed consent* are one thing in general medicine where communication is typically normal, quite another in psychiatric contexts where uneventful or routine communication with disturbed or intellectually impaired patients is more often than not only a clinical dream.

Summarizing: Dr. Cox's results, if viewed as a categorization of ethical issues in the more typical medical services are quite acceptable for both their relevance and comprehensiveness, methodological questions aside. The considerations I have outlined, however, give me reason for believing that the categories leave us at some uncomfortable conceptual distance from the relatively unique and compelling specifics of psychiatric contexts. My other concern, the one I discussed first, is a more formal, philosophical one and stems from the use of socio-empirical data as a primary basis for subsequent analysis. Such an approach tends to fog the technical character of the investigation, making it difficult to decide whether to regard it as a project in normative ethics or in descriptive sociology. How, eventually, to bridge the logical gap from group perceptions to ethical prescriptions remains, therefore, an entirely open question.

Thus, my two concerns are, reduced conceptual pertinence and fact-value confusion. My response to both of them is to favor, for projects of this sort, the researcher's own background of knowledge over episodal data, as the primary grist or basis for reflection and analysis. Ordinarily this is an advanced background spanning both the medical services under consideration and the published body of discourse in medical ethics. Grounded theory strategies can, no doubt, be fruitful in those *de facto* projects where the conceptual and factual background is relatively thin or largely absent. Some sociological areas of inquiry illustrate this very well. Examples would be such topics as, "the personal attitudes towards collusion among financial executives" or "the loneliness of aging American ethnics". But entertaining fresh empirical approaches in ethical inquiry where systematic thinking has its roots in a very long discursive tradition seems to be like asking a theoretical physicist to engage in fresh laboratory experimentation in order to come up with something like the special theory of relativity or a unified field theory. For such purposes, head-on empirical strategies are futile and in actual practice, give way to a mode of theorizing which features reflecting on the existing panorama of fact, concept, paradox, controversy, and *gedanken*-experiments that are never actually carried out. It is this mode of theorizing which has been monumentally productive from Galileo to Einstein. And something very much like it is also the fruitful strategy of choice in ethics and other philosophical areas of human concern where we call it *philosophical analysis*. If I am right about my recommendation, the burden of preliminary data gathering for projects of the kind we are considering can be avoided and research energy channeled to the place where the process of discovery really begins, namely, the reflections of the researcher as she enlivens, broadens, and deepens her insights by shuffling and reshuffling, analyzing, codifying, and interrelating the pertinent facts and concepts already at her command in her own background of knowledge.

NOTE

1. Glaser, B. and Strauss, A. *The Discovery of Grounded Theory:* (Chicago: Aldeen Publishing Co., 1967), pp. 32-35.

ALLOCATION ISSUES AS THEY IMPACT ON THE QUALITY OF LIFE IN HOSPICE CARE

By Margaret Benner and Dorothy Moser
Department of Nursing Science
University of Delaware

Introduction

"Extinction is the fate of species, and death is the fate of each individual human being... Because death is the central, most powerful mystery of human life, it holds profound significance for us all."(1)

It is not death, but rather the quality of life that is central to the hospice philosophy. As an alternative approach to care for the terminally ill, hospice is not a new concept. The word, itself, comes from the Latin root word "hospes," meaning both host and guest, and symbolizing the mutual caring of people for one another. In the Middle Ages, the dying person was thought of as a metaphorical traveler at a stopping place on a long journey that will be continued after death.(2) There was great concern for both the body and the soul. Perhaps it was the recall of that caring attitude for the whole person and an awareness of how far modern medicine had strayed in its phenomenal successes in curing that motivated Cicely Saunders to revive this old concept. She founded the first modern-day hospice (St. Christopher's) in England in the early '60s. Hospice offers an aggressive, caring intervention model for a peaceful and dignified death in place of a medical, cure-oriented model which only emphasizes the failure of medicine and the hopelessness of the dying individual and his/her family.

Hospice came to the United States with the establishment of the Connecticut Hospice in 1974. A little more than a decade later there are literally hundreds of hospice programs in all states all across the nation. They have gained a strong foothold in our health care system and offer a viable option to how one may choose to die from a terminal illness. Care of the terminally ill in the mainstream of health services has had to deal with many ethical issues which have been debated by practitioners and scholars. Questions such as the following have been addressed: 1) Should the patient be told his/her diagnosis/prognosis?; 2) How aggressive should treatment be when medical science really has no cure?; 3) How much pain medication is appropriate for the terminally ill patient?; 4) How long should life be prolonged by artificial means?; 5) Does the patient have the right to refuse/terminate treatment? Within traditional health care institutions, these questions have provoked much debate, ambivalence, and stress among health care workers.

Many of these questions are answered when patients/families opt for hospice care. Within the hospice context a totally honest communications network prevails. No more games are played out. Diagnosis and prognosis are acknowledged. The fact of dying/death is confronted by patient and family with the support of the hospice team of caregivers.

As such, the focus is shifted from treatment and cure to support and care -- from quantity to quality of life. Although the ethical issues which can be identified in hospice care cover a wide spectrum, only those related to allocation of resources will be addressed here. It is not the purpose of this paper to attempt to resolve the issues. Rather, through the use of vignettes, to identify how allocation issues impact on the quality of care provided; and, hence, on the quality of life and/or death. These vignettes are presented and discussed from the perspective of a nurse -- a member of the health care team who has, in the past, been encouraged to follow orders but who, within the hospice movement, finds him or herself in a leadership role.

A number of concerns arise in relation to hospice admission criteria. The first hypothetical case presented here addresses some of those admission issues.

Vignette 1

Mr. & Mrs. J. have lived in a small rural town all their lives. Their childless marriage of fifty-two years has been characterized by unusual closeness. Their happiness has been derived from their shared common interests in their home, garden, and their beloved eleven year old pet poodle. Now, Mr. J. is terminally ill at home. The J's have few financial resources and hospice services will be covered by Medicare.

When they are assessed for hospice admission, it is recognized that they will need a lot of equipment and medications in the home. Mr. J. says that will not be any trouble because they know the local pharmacist and have great trust in him. When hospice investigates, they discover that the local pharmacist charges a lot more for supplies than the pharmacist they usually deal with who gives hospice special rates which are within Medicare guidelines for reimbursement. Mr. and Mrs. J. are requested to obtain their supplies from the hospice-known pharmacist. They flatly refuse, saying they wouldn't trust anyone else and wouldn't feel right taking their business elsewhere. However, they are also adamant about wanting hospice care.

Discussion

This case certainly raises allocation issues. Presently, Medicare reimburses hospice a flat fee per day to cover all costs. This fee is approximately one half that allotted for in-patient care. Any costs over the allocated amount must be absorbed by the hospice. Given this, should the hospice admit Mr. J. knowing they will not receive adequate reimbursement? Because of the extra costs which hospice must absorb, will others be deprived of needed resources? The issue of the "rights" of certain groups and/or individuals to health care is raised. It has been debated whether "health" and/or "health care" are rights; whether monies budgeted for health care ought to be allocated to acute or preventative medicine; which principle of distributive justice is the fairest; and whether more monies ought to be allocated to certain populations or groups.

Certainly these are issues which must concern a nurse both as an individual and as a professional committed to providing quality nursing care to all who need it. However, the more immediate dilemma which faces the nurse, in this situation, arises out of the client advocacy role of nursing. Such an advocacy role, by virtue of nursing's humanistic commitment to the autonomy, self-actualization and development of the patient as a unique individual, goes beyond that of a mere troubleshooter. According to the professional code for nurses, the nurse's primary concern is with the provision of quality nursing care. Thus, the nurse must address at least two questions: 1) Would it be right to deny admission to a patient in need, such as Mr. J., if he/she refuses to go to another pharmacist? and 2) Would the quality of life for Mr. and Mrs. J. be significantly affected by a forced severance of a valued relationship?

The nurse is obligated to assist Mr. J. to die as he chooses as well as to assist him to maintain meaningful positive relationships with other health care providers, such as the pharmacist. The patient has the right to choose his own health care providers as a part of his right to participate in all decisions about his care. Absolutely essential to advocacy is a collaborative relationship. And that demands our consideration of an individual's unique attitudes and feelings. As an advocate, the nurse must act as a coordinator to ensure that the client has "access to all parts of the delivery system that are needed, and that the various services are offered at a time, place, and costs that are reasonable for the client."(3) In this situation, both goals cannot be accomplished and, in fact, conflict unless the pharmacist agrees to lower his prices. If he refuses to do so, the nurse must decide whether to compromise the quality of care provided by attempting to alter a long-standing, positive relationship with another health care provider in order to reduce costs or fight to have Mr. J. admitted to hospice regardless of costs. To do the latter, however, conflicts with a nurse's obligation to help ensure that all citizens' rights to health care are met. If the financial resources of hospice are strained due to absorption of costs, the program may be forced to cease operation or may have to reduce services to others equally in need.

Let us assume that the hospice program, in this case, was able to negotiate with the local pharmacist to reduce his charges, and therefore Mr. J. was admitted to the hospice program. Mrs. J. was able to keep her husband comfortable and to administer medications which kept his pain at a minimum. He was content to die in this atmosphere of love; she was deeply gratified to help him and felt that she'd be sad, but able to live out her life after his death knowing that they had shared these times together. However, that was not to be! Mrs. J. suffered a fatal heart attack, leaving her husband without a primary caregiver, devastated and dying. The closest relative, a great-nephew, lived at a distance and could not offer much help. He felt Mr. J. should go into a nursing home, sell the house, and have the pet poodle put to sleep. Hospice was unable to continue services without a primary caregiver in the home. Mr. J. refused to go to a hospital or nursing home, saying all he wanted was to die in his own home surrounded by his possessions, his beloved pet, and his memories. There was no money for paid help, and the hospice couldn't justify aides under Medicare nor provide the quantity of volunteer help Mr. J. needed. Medically, physicians estimated he could live several months, but was rapidly becoming too weak to care for himself. Should hospice discharge this man? Should they try to get him into a hospital? a nursing home? Or, should they retain him in hospice care?

For the nurse, the issues, once again, revolve around quality of care and patient advocacy. The nurse's multiple loyalties to the hospice, to the individual client, and to other present and future clients present a dilemma. If Mr. J. is retained in the hospice program without a primary caregiver, hospice policy will be violated. Would this be unjust, considering that other clients have been denied admission because there was no primary caregiver? If Mr. J. remains in the hospice program, someone would have to assume the role of primary caregiver. The nurse, acting as client advocate, could attempt to arrange for volunteers, homemakers, aides, or live-in companions to serve in that role. This, however, raises a concern about the quality of care. In this situation, outside employment agencies would have to be relied upon to adequately screen and train personnel. Although these individuals may be technically competent, will they adhere to hospice philosophy, thus assuring Mr. J's right to die as he chooses?

A nurse must assist the client to exercise freedom of choice. If an individual chooses hospice but is refused admission or discharged and, thus, denied the right to die as chosen because there is no primary caregiver, then the client is really not free to choose. Should hospices, thus, be obligated to train and employ all necessary personnel? Should they develop their own in-patient unit for situations such as Mr. J. presents? If hospice should decide to bear the expense of employing outside personnel to care for Mr. J., would this not drain funds and human resources from other families who do meet the criteria for admission? Is it right to admit or retain clients in the program if quality care cannot be provided? If Mr. J. is retained, is it fair to deny admission to other clients who also do not have a primary caregiver? Each has the same need. Is it justifiable to treat clients differently? Because of the covenant relationship, which is a crucial aspect of the hospice program, is there a duty not to abandon care? Has a commitment been made to Mr. J. which cannot now be broken? Even if there is no duty, as a professional who has been trained to "care," can a nurse stop caring and/or stop offering care to a patient in need?

Vignette II

Let us now turn to the issue of the use of hyperalimentation as a treatment modality. Parenteral hyperalimentation or total parenteral nutrition (TPN) is a method of giving highly concentrated solutions intravenously to maintain adequate nutrition. The hospice philosophy emphasizes palliative treatment and control of symptoms. Patients who choose hospice care agree that nothing will be done to prolong life but that pain and suffering will be eased so that death comes as painlessly as possible. As an advocate, the nurse must protect the patient and ensure,

186

as far as possible, that no treatment is performed which violates that commitment.

Consider the following three situations. Is TPN palliative or curative in these cases? Who and how is it decided whether TPN enhances or decreases the quality of life?

Situation 1

Anthony is a one month old infant, sent home from the hospital with multiple congenital anomalies and a predicted life expectancy of one to two months. His mother wishes to offer him love at home as long as he lives and has sought out hospice care. The family has private insurance, but it does not cover the costly TPN treatment that the pediatrician has recommended.

Situation 2

Mary is a twenty-eight year old, severely retarded woman who functions at a three to four year old level. She has always lived with her mother and grandmother who have devoted their lives to the care of this child. Mary's mother is a widow and is on welfare. Mary is terminally ill and is in hospice care. Mary's mother has heard about TPN and wants it for her child, stating that her daughter's only pleasure in life is eating and that she derives great satisfaction from providing nourishment for her. Even though Mary is unable to take food by mouth because of her cancer, the mother cannot bear the thought of not feeding her child. She says, "That's the way I've made her happy all these years and I can't stop now."

Situation 3

Mrs. K. is fifty-six year old woman who prac-ticed law until she had to retire because of cancer of the esophagus. She is married and has two children, a seventeen year old son who will soon graduate from high school and a twenty-one year old daughter who is to be married in two months. Her condition has been rapidly deteriorating, but the physician says that her life expectancy could be extended somewhat with TPN treatment. Mrs. K. says that she could die in peace if she could just live to see her son graduate and her daughter marry.

Discussion

There has been considerable debate within the hospice community as to whether TPN is a palliative or a curative treatment. In a 1984 Ethics Committee survey, many treatments were found to be either ordinary or extraordinary depending on the specific situation.(4) TPN, however, was the only treatment consistently identified as extraordinary and curative. In most instances, TPN is considered to prolong life. However there are situations in which its usage may be considered palliative.

Once again, a dilemma arises for the nurse because of the advocacy role. As an advocate and care coordinator, the nurse is usually the individual who has the most contact with the client and his or her family. It is the nurse's obligation to participate in decision making and to represent the client's interests to ensure that the quality of life and death are maintained. In the three situations presented, is TPN a "good" for the patient as the patient or the proxy decision maker has defined "good"? Would the use of TPN enhance the quality of life and death?

In at least one hospice program the authors know of, a general policy has evolved in which TPN is considered an extraordinary treatment for adults, but a palliative intervention for infants and young children. Although each case is decided on an individual basis, the rationale is that nurturing and love are not as intimately associated with feeding in the case of adults as with infants or young children. That is, the child (and perhaps the retarded adult also) receives nurturing and love primarily through feeding and its accompanying physical contact. Likewise, parents give nurturing and love to their children primarily through feeding and its accompanying physical contact to their infants. Adults, on the other hand, have other means of giving and receiving nurturing and love. But, is this rationale justified?

Is it right to make different decisions based on either chronological or mental age? If it is considered evil in the hospice view to prolong life but a positive goal to decrease suffering, would not the Principle of Double Effect permit the use of TPN to alleviate suffering even though its usage prolongs life? Amenta states that the contemporary criteria is becoming the usefulness or benefit of the treatment to the patient, not the treatment per se, and that there is a duty to "...sustain life by means that do not put patient or family at undue burden relative to the benefit received."(5) In the case of the infant, does the mother benefit from the fulfillment of her nurturing needs even if the infant's dying process is prolonged by TPN? Even if the use of TPN is justifiable, it is an extremely expensive procedure which requires professional monitoring. Again the question arises, is it fair to expend this amount of money and human resources for TPN if it means less are available for other hospice patients who do not need this intervention?

Summary

Dilemmas for the nurse, in all these cases, arise because of conflict within the advocacy role. Although hospice care utilizes a multidisciplinary approach, Medicare requirements mandate that nurses assume a leadership role by acting as the team care plan coordinator. The care received determines, to a large degree, the peace and dignity with which death is approached. "Care, comfort, help for pain, protection during illness, encouragement and support, hope and humane concern are all immediate values arising from the nurse-patient relationship."(6) The clinician's strong sense of obligation to individual patients and families will always clash with the program's need to economize. Nurses have an obligation to participate in formulating public policy. This arises out of an obligation to individual patients. The system may continue "as is" because nurses have not always fought to change it. Nursing is the largest group of health care providers and, as such, can be very influential if they exercise their collective responsibility.

Acting as a coordinator of hospice care does not mean that the nurse knows any more, ethically. But, it does obligate the nurse, at the very least, to actively contribute as an equal participant on the team in ethical decision making. Regardless of the nurse's role on the health care team, he/she must be concerned with moral decision making. Yet, more often than not, nurses have not been educationally prepared to engage, systematically, rather than intuitively, in moral reasoning.

As hospice care expands in this country, what is to prevent it from compromising the ethical principles upon which it was founded? Some potential safeguards do exist for the perpetuation of ethical practice in hospice care. One of these is the inherent multidisciplinary team approach to care. Cassidy suggests that the team power for decision making may, indeed, be the most ethical strategy for preservation of quality of life for the terminally ill and their families. He thinks that the team can best address dilemmas because it includes both the "authentic voice" of the patient/family unit (an extreme autonomous perspective) and knowledgeable, experienced professionals/volunteers (an extreme heteronomous perspective).(7) Rather than abhorring conflict, Cassidy advocates promoting/respecting conflict in order to make "good" ethical decisions. He recommends the "...respect for the otherness of others" which he reminds us is Buber's definition of love.(8) To further the team decision-making power, a preventative ethics program or ethical rounds ought to be a critical component of hospice team deliberations. This allows for planned opportunities to debate ethical dilemmas in an unharassed setting and also provides for different disciplines/cultures to see how each views difficult situations related to death/dying.

Another safeguard for ethical practice in hospice care lies in the honest/open communications channels which are inherent in its philosophy. These promote decision making which is both within the legal boundaries of society and personal values boundaries of the specific individuals involved in a dilemma.

Deliberations within such a context, combined with continuously developing expertise in the ethical decision-making process, hold great potential for competency in the resolution of recurring and new ethical dilemmas which occur in hospice care.

It is the impression of the authors of this paper that hospice families/personnel will not only develop their expertise in ethical resolutions, but that they can significantly influence the entire health care system by serving as models for coping with ethical issues in all health care settings. What a challenging and exciting opportunity!

REFERENCES

1. Amenta, Madalon O'Rowe and Nancy L. Bohnet. *Nursing Care of the Terminally Ill* (Boston: Little, Brown & Co., 1986), p. 21.
2. Stoddard, Sandol. *The Hospice Movement: A Better Way of Caring for the Dying* (N.Y.: Vintage Books, 1978).
3. Leddy, Susan and J. Mae Pepper. *Conceptual Bases of Professional Nursing* (Philadelphia: J.B. Lippincott Company, 1985), p. 286.
4. Mishkin, B. and Arras, J. *Ethical Perspectives for Hospice Care Givers.* Annual Meeting and Symposium of the National Hospice Organization, Hartford, CN, Nov. 11, 1984.
5. Amenta, *op. cit.*, p. 338.
6. Jameton, Andrew. *Nursing Practice: The Ethical Issues* (Englewood Cliffs, New Jersey: Prentice Hall, 1984), p. 238.
7. Cassidy, Robert C. "Ethical Issues in Team Conflict." Staff Development Presentation to Delaware Hospice, Wilmington, DE, February 18, 1987.
8. *Ibid.*

THE DEFEASIBILITY AND LIMITS
OF RIGHTS TO HOSPICE CARE
Reply to Professors Benner and Moser

By Susan Rae Peterson
Nassau Community College

The first issue raised by the very thoughtful and morally sensitive paper presented here by Margaret Benner and Dorothy Moser concerning moral problems and dilemmas in hospice care is one concerning the ethics of the *philosophical reply*. There are several standard and acceptable approaches in giving replies to conference papers, e.g., analysis and rebuttal using philosophical terminology, a first-order normative discussion of the moral issues actually raised by the paper, and so forth. An entirely philosophical reply would be unsatisfactory to laypersons and medical personnel, and an entirely un-philosophical reply would amount to no more than a sharing of personal views on medical moral issues. I call this problem one of the applied ethics of doing applied ethics. My solution is to focus upon two philosophical concepts in ethics, moral rights and their *prima facie* nature, which make them defeasible by other moral considerations -- to answer directly some of the moral questions raised by Benner and Moser. These familiar moral concepts should facilitate a sound reasoning process with which to solve real and recurring problems in medical ethics occurring within the hospice environment.

Benner and Moser identify the moral crux of the issue at hand to be medical resource allocation; however, I believe it is the conflict between the patients' rights and the professionals' rights. Naturally, with an infinite amount of medical resources, none of these moral problems would arise. However, since the American medical situation continues to make medical care scarce, we must simply assume that many deserving patients will have to forego desirable (or even necessary) care, and therefore that medical professionals -- especially nurses in the hospice example -- will have to bear the burden of making difficult choices. In fact, many of the moral dilemmas presented by Benner and Moser are instances of triage, i.e., making choices in life-or-death situations as to who shall be treated and who shall not. Given the seriousness of such decisions, it would seem to be an absolute necessity for hospices to institute formalized procedures for moral decision making to assist the professionals making these decisions.

Although there are various views about rights in the philosophical community (in which debates continue to rage), few would challenge the claim that rights are *prima facie*, that is, they exist *ceteris paribus*, other things being equal, but may under certain conditions be overridden by other factors. My right to free speech is limited by public safety, and so can be overridden by such a factor (yelling "Fire!" in a crowded theatre, when there is no fire, is not within my rights). In triage cases, although every victim has a right to be cared for and saved, it is frequently the case that only some *can* be saved, and so some people's rights may be overridden by a concern for saving as many as possible. For example, the medication problems of Mr. J., who wishes to use his own pharmacist, can be resolved once we understand the extent and the defeasibility of his rights and the nurse's duty to the patient. Although Mr. J. does have a right to hospice care he presumably does not have a right to dictate hospice policy on the reimbursement of pharmacy costs. Moreover, it is not clear that denying Mr. J. his choice of pharmacists would seriously affect his quality of life. The patient's right to autonomy, like other rights, is not absolute; in other words, it does not extend to the point of obligating others to satisfy his goals and desires. Naturally, if many or most of Mr. J.'s desires concerning his own care were ignored by medical personnel, his autonomy would in fact be threatened. A decision, for example, concerning whether or not the patient ought to take any drugs, or how much, etc., would much more affect his autonomy than would the matter of *who* provides his medication. Also, there are other solutions: (1) ask Mr. J.'s pharmacist for special rates; (2) have Mr. and Mrs. J. reimburse the hospice for the difference in rates; (3) ask Mr. J.'s pharmacist to supervise his medications provided by another pharmacist. Medical professionals in the hospice do not have a duty to provide care to him in *all* matters *only* as he would wish. Surely the moral consideration of ceasing to be a client of a pharmacist is insignificant compared to losing hospice care.

Although there is always a difficulty in assessing each situation and the moral ramifications of various courses of action, the patient's autonomy must be protected *within* the context of the medical program involved. Of course, I am assuming that the policies of the hospice have been developed in an overall just manner, for the benefit of the patients in general. Given this, there is nothing morally wrong in adhering to these policies, since, as Benner and Moser admit, violating hospice policies may well deprive other patients of their deserved treatment. (It goes without saying that in any given case which is created by an unjust medical policy, the moral solution to the problem may well be changing the hospice policy.)

The hospice policy in the pharmacy example appears to me just; it ought not be extended or violated just because Mr. J. wishes to remain with his own pharmacist. In the matter of trust, perhaps some trust ought to be transferred from his previous health care provider to the new hospice staff. The *prima facie* nature of rights, as well as the *ceteris paribus* clause attaching to all moral principles, best explains my resolution of the problem. The resulting situation when Mrs. J. dies, however, presents a different and more serious problem. It is perhaps unavoidable in hospices to face continual problems of turning down needy applicants based on factors concerning the family's ability to care at home for the patient. The very nature of the hospice makes this factor a necessary ingredient in any moral decision. Unfortunately, hospices (non-hospital bed hospices at any rate) cannot afford, nor were ever intended to afford, providing total health care in the absence of family or home members. The mere desire on behalf of a patient to die at home *with* hospice care, when the circumstances preclude the possibility of the hospice providing such care, does not constitute an absolute right, or even a weaker right, on behalf of the patient. The patient *does* have the right to refuse treatment in general, however. The only recourse left to the hospice nurse, her professional duty because of the medical care relationship already created within the hospice environment, would be to persuade the patient to seek care in a hospital or nursing home. Should the patient refuse, he has a legal and moral right to die at home without medical care. The hospice, however, would exceed its justifiable charter by providing hospital care or other in-patient care to a patient who does not satisfy the criteria for a hospice patient in the first place.

The problem at hand is nonetheless interesting, i.e., determining the proper extent of duty to the patient based on past treatment after he or she has ceased to qualify for treatment. All one can say in this brief reply is that the parameters of hospice care and its corresponding moral commitments to patients should always be made very explicit both to patients and staff, so that recognizing the boundaries becomes less problematic all around. The hospice staff, ultimately, cannot force Mr. J. not to die "as chosen" since he retains the right to refuse any and all treatment and may therefore die alone in his home if he wishes. To leave room for discussion, I shall only comment briefly on TPN, a problem attractive to philosophers because it involves the possibility of providing for life extension *and* a palliation for suffering. The philosophical and moral resolution that TPN raises, however, is quite standard, given the moral principles involved. As Benner and Moser explain, the paramount goal in hospice care is to allow terminal patients to die with dignity and in comfort; they claim, almost casually, that this requires the further condition that "nothing will be done to prolong life." Now this surely overstates the *prima facie* duties of the hospice's health care professional staff, for certainly they are not trying to *shorten* the lives of their patients. Indeed, if this last priority were taken seriously, then anything (such as TPN) that had the dual effect of prolonging life and diminishing suffering would be prohibited in a hospice, since prolonging life would be considered wrong. However, my philosophical approach can resolve this apparent dilemma: Only when TPN is used for the explicit purpose of prolonging life, to the detriment of the general condition of the patient, would its use be wrong. Thus, the mother in the case study *should* receive TPN because her quality of life would be greatly enhanced to see her son graduate and her daughter marry.

Moser and Benner ask if it is right to make different decisions based on age, either mental or chronological. Yes, it is morally right to do so, in cases where age is morally relevant. Medical decisions are frequently made on such grounds, and properly so, such as in triage cases: when only some can be saved, it is better to save the young rather than the old. The facts of human existence (e.g., that we suffer, that we have a given life expectancy, that only women bear children, etc.) are what give rise to morality in the first place, and so it is not surprising that such facts are relevant in moral decision-making. (Of course, age *may* be entirely irrelevant in certain cases, as when a 20-year old and a 22-year old require a new kidney.) In the case of the mother of the severely retarded 28-year-old woman, the mother's need to provide nourishment weighs only slightly against the health risks this presents to her daughter. The mother's right is negligible here, given the specific circumstances described. It would not be fair, then, to spend the money and human resources for TPN in cases in which there are counterbalancing moral and medical factors, and which would result in less care for future patients *without* such counter-balancing factors.

To end on a practical note, let me make a suggestion. Perhaps the hospice health care team could institute formal procedures for making moral decisions in the institution. The best way would be to use examples such as presented in Benner and Moser's paper, discuss the various principles involved in the case, and then try to explicate as clearly as possible the deliberation process of the group. Of course, in cases of moral dilemmas, i.e., cases in which no matter which action one takes one moral principle or another is violated, some wrong will result. However, this is just a fact of life, and is not restricted to health care decisions. What is needed are formal procedures to buttress the fortitude of the health care team so that they can implement such decisions with as much support as possible.

MORALITY AND LEGALITY OF NIGERIAN TRADITIONAL MEDICAL THERAPY

By H.O.T. Ajala
Research Fellow II
National Institute for Medical Research
Yaba - Lagos, Nigeria

Acknowledgement

I would like to thank the Director and staff of the National Institute for Medical Research (N.I.M.R.) where I work as a Research Fellow for sponsoring the trip to attend this unique conference on "Professional Ethics on Healing Arts." I am grateful to its supervising Ministry, the Federal Ministry of Science and Technology, for giving its approval to present my paper.
I would sincerely from the bottom of my heart like to thank the organizers of this conference -- the Long Island Philosophical Society, particularly its Chairman in the person of Dr. Eugene Kelly, who has facilitated my stay in New York, to present my paper by helping me to get a grant to cover the accommodation expenses while I am attending this unique conference.
I am grateful to both the President and his Public Relations Officer of Nigerian Council of Traditional Medicine Practitioners for the co-operation given for making this paper possible. I am grateful to the Legal adviser of the Nigerian Alternative Medical Association (NAMA) Chief Afe Babalola SAN (Senior Advocate of Nigeria.
Finally, I am indebted to Dr. E.A. Adegoke, Associate Professor, Department of Chemistry, University of Lagos, for his assistance in the preparation of this paper.

INTRODUCTION

It gives me great pleasure to be here today for this unique conference titled "PROFESSIONAL ETHICS IN THE HEALING ARTS" organized by Long Island Philosophical Society. Before I come to the main theme of my paper, "Morality and Legality of Nigerian Traditional Medical Therapy," I would like to state that the relationship between medicine and the rest of the culture has been noted by Ackerknecht,(1942) who said, "Medicine is nowhere independent and following its own motivations. Its character and dynamism depend on the place it takes in every cultural pattern; they depend on the pattern itself".

Concepts of diseases are cultural classifications of adversity. They do not of course cover the whole range of misfortune a society may face. The early scientists accepted what people called the essential elements like air, water, earth and fire. These elements were used for their comfort and welfare. Other substances and materials such as vegetation and animal, in addition to the already mentioned elements, were used. All these have been used for human needs. Vegetation gives us food, and serves as sources of medical concoctions if applied in time of illness and in the treatment of diseases. The frequent use of various herbs, plants, leaves, roots, and minerals in the treatment of the sick became a tradition which was handed down from one generation to another over the years. Thus, Nigerian traditional medical therapy developed and traditional physicians gained their knowledge through experience in the practice of this science of treatment of the sick.

Traditional Medicine is an art, science, philosophy and practice that follows definite natural, biological, chemical, mental and spiritual laws for the restoration and maintenance of health and the correction of bodily disorders. Traditional Medicine makes use of nature's inherent powers and the use of its agencies is based on the theory that under natural conditions of normal living the body in its environment is a self-healing organism.

The traditional medical doctor is not restricted to any particular part of the world, nor to any tribe or race. As a matter of fact, traditional physicians have always been part of any community, be it advanced or developing. In developed countries like the United States of America and Canada, the development of science education and advancement in technology have paved the way for recognition of chiropractic medicine and other natural medical sciences. The evolution of modern medical therapy is the result of the systematic and scientific investigation of medicinal plants which formed the bulk of the ingredients of the prescriptions of traditional health practitioners. The evaluation of the extractives of these medicinal plants gives useful information about their physiological activity, which is in turn applied in medical therapy.

In a developing country like Nigeria, efforts are currently being made in the scientific investigation of medicinal plants. The majority of the people in Nigeria irrespective of their class and social status still use herbs and attend the clinics of traditional medical doctors when they are sick. In Nigeria, facilities of well-equipped giant hospitals built and staffed with allopathic medical specialists are available, but yet the majority of the Nigerian people both in the rural and urban areas prefer to go to Nigerian traditional healers. However, we should not also forget that in advanced countries, such as the United Kingdom and the United States of America, with their modern hospitals, herbal shops, health food stores, and herbal clinics also flourish and enjoy a large patronage.

In Nigeria, as in most parts of Africa, the traditional physician has in the past been called a native doctor. The word "native," as used by the former colonial masters, has a derogatory under-tone. The native physician was regarded as a juju man, magician or witch-doctor. This campaign of hate went on for many years, but still the native medical doctor enjoys up to the present date a wide patronage of his or her people living in the same community. His clinic is usually full of patients who have implicit faith in his ability to diagnose their ailments and give efficacious prescriptions of natural remedies. As a Research Fellow of the National Institute for Medical Research, Yaba - Lagos, Nigeria and a National Executive Secretary of Nigerian Alternative Medical Association (NAMA), I am fully aware of the popularity of Nigerian traditional healers. I sincerely believe that the time has come for the scientific investigation and study of the extractives of the medicinal plants which form the basis of the medical prescriptions used by the traditional doctors. Before embarking on this study, I had already realized the need to enjoy the confidence and co-operation of traditional doctors in order to achieve any progress in this direction.

I feel comfortable in saying that we in the division of Pharmacology and Therapeutics at the National Institute for Medical Research, Yaba - Lagos have succeeded in winning the confidence of Nigerian traditional doctors because many of them had come to our institute with various medicinal plants, roots leaves, and minerals, for the treatment of various diseases. We have been able to make a compilation of these medicinal plants. We also get a continual flow of valuable information from them in regard to their prescriptions and the production of the authentic ingredients which make up these prescriptions.

In order to secure full cooperation with Nigerian traditional doctors in our research, I was permitted by the Director of the Institute to meet some prominent members of the Traditional Medicine Association, even in their houses.

My meeting with them had instilled confidence in them for displaying to me the various types of medicinal herbs they have. They have since come to discuss at our Institute the nature, mechanics, and methodology of their practice. In addition, they had the opportunity to exchange views and ideas with modern medical specialists and scientists, who, because of their scientific background and training, will be able to analyze critically and objectively such information as may be provided by the traditional doctors. The objective of both the traditional and modern doctor is the same, which is to maintain the health of the people. It is the mechanics, methodology, and philosophy which differ. But even then there are bound to be areas of similarity which can be usefully developed such that the traditional method can be complementary to the modern. My findings are supported by the fact that in countries like India and China, traditional and modern hospitals function in cooperation with each other and are inter-dependent, thus giving the patient every facility that is humanly possible in medical attention.

Since independence, Nigeria has started to provide modern health services for her people under the leadership of Prof. Olukoyo Ransome-Kuti, the Hon. Minister of Health and his predecessor Dr. E. Nsan. But the lack of finances in developing countries including Nigeria might make this provision of modern health service unrealistic at the appropriate time -- by the year 2000, the World Health Organization (WHO) projection. The main cause of the inadequacies in health care services in Nigeria is that her pattern of medical care and education of health personnel were copied closely from the Western countries, particularly Britain, France, and the United States of America; and yet these advanced countries have changed to a more realistic approach to total health by recognizing alternative medicine such as Chiropractic, Homeopathy, Osteopathy, Acupuncture and Naturopathy and Herbalism. Nigeria is fully ready to imbibe these patterns, for they are very relevant to the needs of the developing countries like Nigeria.

ETHNOMEDICAL THERAPY

Therapy in traditional medicine is a vast subject. It includes both magico-religions and mechanical and chemical procedures. Laughlin (1963) has made the point that the success of the human species is in no small measure due to its ability to cope with medical problems: an assessment of indigenous medical systems, including those of literate societies, shows an impressive array of practices that demonstrate empirical therapeutic knowledge including trephining, bone-setting, removal of ovaries, obstetrics including laparotomy, uvulectomy, cautery, inoculation baths, poultices, inhalations, laxatives, enema, ointments, and cupping (Ackerknecht 1942, Simmons 1955, Laughlin 1963, Huard 1969). The pharmacopoeia of traditional medicine is copious and includes such proven remedies.

When illness occurs. it is either ignored or treated without consultation of a specialist (Polgar 1962).

When a patient consults a health practitioner for the treatment of a certain disease, other specialists are usually involved e.g., traditional gynecologists or obstetricians. Therapists may specialize in only one type of skill or they may combine several in their practice (Liebau 1962). Prof. Lambo (Deputy Director General of the World Health Organization) finds that some traditional health practitioners are very good, and that a lot of benefits can be gained from their wealth of knowledge. He made this remark at a pre-one year anniversary Conference of *Health Care Magazine*. He stated that he had picked twelve traditional health practitioners to work with him at Neuro-Psychiatric Hospital, Aro - Abeokuta, Ogun State, Nigeria, as reported in the *Daily Times,* Wednesday, February 18th, 1987.

TRAINING

Qualification for traditional medical systems vary considerably. In most cases, no formal training may be required for practitioners (Metzger and Williams, 1963), while in others an apprenticeship may be customary (Maclean 1969).

The bone setter specialist exists in every ethnic group in Nigeria. Yoruba bone setters are well noted for their accurate diagnosis and treatment of frac-tured bones (Oyebola 1980). Once the diagnosis of fracture is made, the traditional bone setter starts with careful manipulation of the bone. He realigns the affected bone. He then applies a hot fermenta-tion of a herbal concoction. Herbal lotion is applied, and then the affected limb is bandaged and splinted with pieces of raffia woven into a sheet big enough to wrap round the affected limb. This procedure is carried out twice daily -- morning and night until the fractured bone has united. The patient is then gradually made mobile by using wooden crutches.

However, not all traditional remedies can be subjected to test tube evaluation, e.g., treatments involving the case of amulets, medicinal rings, incantations and sacrifices. The African tradition of health cannot all be explained on the basis of pharmacological activities. Limbs crippled by arthritis, leg ulcers, nervous troubles, bronchitis, urinary difficulties, skin disease, and both female and male diseases are just a few disorders which have responded very successfully to herbal medication.

REMEDY PREPARATION

Traditional health practitioners and pharmacists prepare their remedies by pounding with a mortar or grinding with stone all the components together. Others are made by the pounding of leaf and boiling of the remaining leaf to form a concoction. Some are dried and pulverized into a powder. In brief, grinding, pulverizing and drying form the main methods of traditional medicine preparation and extraction is the main chemical process involved.

REMEDY ADMINISTRATION

There are mainly two ways of administering remedies, namely

1. Oral administration;
2. External application through the skin.

The oral administration could involve a liquid or a powder mixed with pap, palm wine or any other food.

The following medicinal plants have offered alternatives for the treatment of diseases which otherwise would involve modern combative operations for many patients, especially for those who are poor and live in rural areas far away from hospitals.

HERBAL TREATMENT

	Disease	Treatment	How Given
1.	Infective hepatitis	Bark of alstonia; Congensis in palm wine	Oral
2.	Sickle cell disease	Alcoholic extract of the root of fagara xanthacyloids	Oral
3.	Rheumatism; black blood disease	Aqueous extract of the root of clausene anisata	Oral
4.	Back Pain	Aqueous extract of the leaves of chasmanthera dependens	Oral
5.	Hypopigmented rashes	Aqueous extract of the leaves of acapypha ciliata	Oral
6.	Peripheral rashes	Aqueous extract of the root of vernonia cenerea	Oral
7.	Fractured bone	Warm extract of the root of chasomonthera dependens	External
8.	Caesarian Sectional operation	Warm daily bath with the leaves of ceratotheca sesamoid	External
9.	Cholera	Leaves of ocimum gratissimum	Oral
10.	Malaria	Leaves of morinda lucida or rauwolfia vomitoria	Oral

11.	Whooping Cough	Juice of pycnanthus senegalensis or costus ofer	Oral
12.	Gonorrhea, Schistosomiasis	Leaves of ficus exasperata	Oral
13.	Maternity and Infant Care		
	a. to keep fetus healthy and growing	Leaves of hybanthus enneaspermum	Oral
	b. to ease delivery	Leaves of hybanthus enneaspermum	Oral
	c. to minimize teething pains	Leaves of alternanthera repens	Oral
	d. to help toddlers	Leaves of daniella oliveri	Oral
14.	To expel worms	Roots of spigelia anthelmia	External
15.	Ulcers	Bark of enantia chloranta	External
16.	Boils	Leaves of pergularia extensa	External
17.	Conjunctivitis	Heliotroium indicum	External
18.	To control Diabetes	Hunteria umbellata	
19.	Cancer	Morinda lucida, annona senegalensis, poteriem soinosium	
20.	Hypertension	Roots and leaves of spephania	

CHEMICAL CONSTITUENTS OF THE MEDICINAL PLANTS

Chemists, pharmacognosists, pharmacists, nutritionists and modern doctors in different disciplines in Nigerian universities and medical research institutes put a lot of effort into analyzing chemotherapeutic ingredients of our medicinal plants. While it is very important to know the chemical components of every reported medicinal plant, it is equally important that botanists and other scientists whose work is connected with plants should make permanent records of the knowledge of the traditional doctors who gave out the knowledge. Most faculties of pharmacy in Nigerian universities and the Public Health Division at the National Institute for Medical Research where I work as a Research Fellow have become involved in the work of traditional doctors. A list of the Nigerian herbs is being screened with a view to fueling scientific evidence for the efficacy of Nigerian medicinal herbs.

As said earlier, infective hepatitis, a variety of jaundice, has no permanent orthodox medical treatment. The patient is simply confined to bed and is placed on glucose drinks. An oral application of the palm wine extract of the bark of Alstonia Congenensis effects a permanent cure within a few days. No lasting treatment of sickle cell disease has been achieved by the orthodox use of antibiotics. But the traditional use of fagara zanthoxyloides has brought relief to patients suffering from this disease. The orthodox doctor has no problem in treating rheumatism, one of the so-called "black blood" diseases. It is disputable whether osteomyelitis, another "black blood" disease can also be effectively treated at the early stage.

Allopathic orthodox therapy also fails in the treatment of back-ache when there is no determined cause after X-ray examination, clinical test on history or even serum examination, and the traditional doctor has succeeded in treating this type of problem by giving his patient to drink an aqueous extract of the leaves of chasmanthera dependens. Also the traditional healer has succeeded in treating cases of peripheral neuritis which has resisted orthodox medical therapy by application of an extract of the root vernonia cenerea. ("Studies of Nigerian Medicinal Plants: Efficacy and Chemical Constituents." A. Akinsanya & E.A. Adegoke, 1973.)

It might be of interest to know how successful and effective is the application of Nigerian medicinal plants as a substitute for the treatment of ailments and diseases, which in allopathic orthodox therapy involves a combative approach, such as a surgical procedure. In the traditional approach, the treatment of fractured bones is accomplished by the external application of a warm extract of the leaves of chasmanthera dependens. Caesarian sectional operations, when necessitated by narrow pelvis measurement, is often avoided by a daily bath of virginia in a warm concoction containing mainly the leaf of ceratotheca sesamoid.

ANTI-CANCER AGENTS

Cancer, as we all know, is one of the major killer diseases and presently is causing a lot of psychological problems for all mankind. Because of this, the plant kingdom is receiving special attention from health researchers, particularly cancer researchers, who hope to find tumor-inhibiting agents in nature that can provide prototypes for the synthesis of anti-cancer chemicals. The current thinking in the drug industry is that naturally-derived drugs could be safer and more effective. Moreover, plants should be regarded as high-value natural resources. It was reported in *The Guardian* of July 2nd., 1985 (one of the Nigerian daily newspapers) that catharautus roseus (Rose Periwinkle), whose extract is effective against leukemia, is becoming rare because of its high commercial value. World-wide sales of the remedies are in excess of N100 million.

An investigation into Nigerian plants such as annona senegalensis, poterium spinosum, and morinda lucida have yielded promising results in the struggle against cancer. The crystalline material isolated from the plants' parts have been shown to exhibit carcinostatic effect on cancer cells in vitro. (Durodola 1974, 1975, 1976: B)

ANTI-INFECTIVE AGENTS

1.   Aceratum conyzoides is commonly used in Nigeria for wound and ulcer dressings. Adesogun and Okunade (1978, 1979) isolated and characterized pure materials which were tested on artificially created wounds to test their anti-bacterial activity. It was found that the plant is active against micro-organism (staphylococcus nureus in particular), and it was found superior to what is used as lately as 1979 in our modern conventional hospitals for treating burns. The compound was named conyz gerin.

2.   Zanthoxlum zanthonyloides (fagara zanthoxyloids) X-zanthoxyloides is another major plant species, whose roots are used as chewing sticks in Nigeria. The powdered root materials have been found effective for the treatment of oral ailments. Odebiyi and Sofowora (1979) isolated and identified anti-bacterial agents from the roots of X-zanthoxyloides. The finding confirmed that its alkaloid contains anti-sickle cell and anti-microbial agents.

WHAT A PROSPECTIVE PATIENT SHOULD LOOK FOR IN CHOOSING A TRADITIONAL DOCTOR

Cleanliness should always be first observed in the surrounding of a traditional doctor. The traditional health practitioner must be consistent. Patients must be given advice that smoking and the drinking of alcohol are not good. The patient is also advised to vaccinate his children.

The traditional doctor has at his disposal a complete range of natural remedies and it is noteworthy to see orthodox medicine now accepting certain principles and treatments which have been used by the traditional doctors for a long time.

A vital requirement in any healer is absolute honesty. No profit is gained by hiding from a patient the true nature of his or her disorder. When a case history of the disease is fully discussed with the patient concerned, together with the treatments and the reasons for them, the full co-operation of the patient is achieved.

The patient himself becomes involved in his treatment which then becomes more effective. When a satisfactory course of treatment has been established, it is necessary that the patient continue with same traditional doctor as far as possible. No lasting benefit can be gained from changing physicians, as a new course of treatment would have to be started and a fresh relationship built up. No two individuals are exactly the same. In other words, individuals as well as disorders respond in different ways to treatment. The record shows that some patients show a very quick response while others need a long period for a full cure. Hope should never be given up by a patient, because some disorders appear to get worse before improving, and sometimes symptoms sometimes alter during the course of treatment. Under such circumstances, the value of the practitioners can be estimated and appreciated.

INTEGRATION

Traditional medical practitioners now practice openly alongside of the orthodox doctor. Both traditional and modern doctors have same objective. This is in effect the maintenance of the good health of the people. Interestingly enough, a greater number of the populace depends on traditional medicine for healthcare, success in business, in work, commerce, games, sports, examinations love, and home and family life, to name just a few. The science behind its practice, however, remains unknown to most Nigerian allopathic orthodox doctors (Baiyole, 198). However, traditional medical practitioners and orthodox medical practitioners differ widely in the philosophy and in the scope and method of their practice. They both remain content with their own philosophy. Whereas the scope of practice of the orthodox doctor is limited to the physical realm, that of traditional doctors is based both on physical and non-physical realms. This might be the reason why physical science alone might not be a sufficient explanation of why a greater number of the populace depends on traditional medicine for health care. Generally, both the traditional and the modern doctor are concerned for the improvement of the community's health and they make a genuine effort to cure and prevent diseases in order to maintain good health. For such common objectives to be meaningful, the two groups should put their resources together. In Nigeria, the integration of the two is necessary since eighty percent of the population lives in the rural areas and depends on the more readily available and cheaper facilities of traditional medicine. The health consumers consider the two as inevitable partners in the improvement of their health conditions. They find the role of both groups complementary. The health consumers therefore find themselves in two worlds which are not mutually exclusive -- the traditional and modern health practitioners' worlds.

By trial and error in their quest for mental, physical, social, emotional, and psychological well-being, the health consumers have identified what particular cases they would usually refer to traditional practitioners. Therefore, they move freely between the two groups in their efforts to solve their health problems. The co-existence of both the modern and traditional practitioners offers a psychological support to the health consumer who might have otherwise been frustrated, despondent, disillusioned, and thrown out of gear if he has had to depend, without a sure alternative, solely on one consultant who may not always be available and accessible, or who may be failing him. To the patient, then, the co-existence of all types of health personnel leaves no room for any vacuum in his life and in his ever constant craving for care in all its complex ramifications in his local native environment.

But for the sake of humanity and health consumers alone, the need is urgent for a realistic exploration and appraisal of the problems and prospects of legitimating and integrating aspects of traditional health care systems and methods of operation with modern therapy.

WAYS TO INCREASE HEALTH MANPOWER IN NIGERIA

1.   Reorganization of all health personnel.

2. Training of traditional physicians in modern medicine, particularly in how to deliver maternal and child health care, family planning, and public health services.
3. Education for more physicians, nurses and other health personnel.
4. Training for other non-professionals to do some of what physicians do.

NIGERIAN LAW ON MEDICAL AND DENTAL PRACTITIONERS: ACT OF 1963

The Medical and Dental Practitioners Act 1963, Section 14 (Offenses) states as follows:

1. Subject to sub-sections (6) and (7) of this section, if any person who is not a fully registered medical practitioner:
   (a) for or in expectation of reward holds himself out to practice as a medical practitioners; or
   (b) takes or uses any of the following titles, that is to say physician, surgeon, doctor or licentiate of medicine, medical practitioner or apothecary; or
   (c) without reasonable excuse takes or uses any name, title, addition or description implying that he is authorized by law to practice as medical practitioners, he shall be guilty of an offence.

So says the Nigerian Law on Medical and Dental Practitioners' Act of 1963. This Act of 1963 sounds very good because that law does not preclude others qualified doctors or physicians from practicing their own brand of medicine.

As a matter of fact, sub-section six (6) of the same section fourteen expressly provides that what is said in section fourteen has no application to other groups of medical practitioners including Nigerian traditional healers. It reads thus: "where any person is acknowledged by the members generally of the

213

community to which he belongs as having being trained on a system of the therapeutics traditionally in use in that community nothing in paragraph (a) of sub-section (1) shall be construed as making it an offence for that person to practice or to hold himself to practice that system."

This means in effect that those who practice Nigerian traditional medicine and other alternative medicines, such as osteopathy, chiropractic, homeopathy and acupuncture have been recognised by the government of Nigeria since 1963.

It also indicates that before the eyes of the law and the courts all forms of healing practitioners are practicing medicine and as such they should be regarded as medical practitioners and physicians regardless of the branch, system, and method of medicine they are permitted to practice.

In view of the foregoing, what is now needed in order to attain total health care for all by the year 2000 are:

(a)   A constructive attitude towards all forms of healing professions;
(b)   All practitioners of healing arts, traditional and modern doctors should pool their intellectual efforts and financial resources and unite positively in an educational and legislative programme for the greatest good of the greatest number, and to grant the same rights and liberties to all lay individuals and groups of adult age and who are of sound mind to make a choice.

For instance, the Nuremberg war criminal trials in 1947 judged the Nazi doctors, who carried out sadistic experiments, to have acted against accepted values of humanity. This set the stage for a new phase of healing ethics in medical ethics in which the autonomy of the patient became the central focus. It is interesting that the Nuremberg court was reinforcing a principle which had been enunciated by a prominent American jurist, Justice Cardozo, in 1914: "Every human being of adult years and sound mind has a right to determine what shall be done with his own body." (Schloendo H. versus Society of New York Hospital, 105 N.E. 92, 93 [N.Y. 1914]. Ethics has been a fundamental concern to the practice of medicine in all ages, but its rapid rise as a subject of interest in medicine, in medical research, in law, in the social sciences, philosophy and religion, is a phenomenon of the post World-War II period. In earlier ages, medical ethics dealt with the obligations and responsibilities of the physician. The principal concern of the doctor for the welfare of his patient and the clear admonishment to do no harm were embodied in the Hippocratic Oath and all subsequent medical codes. All of these statements of ethics were professionally oriented.

IN VIEW OF THE FOREGOING, WHO THEN CAN HELP

The growth of traditional medicine throughout the country has been rapid. Traditional medicine is neither in opposition nor at variance with allopathic orthodox medicine, surgery or any other system of medicine. As with banning racial discrimination world-over, the time is equally ripe to eliminate discrimination among the health practitioners, whether it be a case of a doctor of allopathic orthodox medicine, chiropractic, osteopathy, of the homeopathic-physician, acupuncturist, or the traditional doctor. In my opinion, in building a solid good house, many artisans are needed: the architect, the carpenters, electricians, plumbers, painters, and sometimes a landscape gardener. The work of each does not duplicate, it complements the others, and all together complete the structure.

People who are afraid to accept a certain type of treatment because it is unusual or unfashionable are entitled to their opinions, of course. On the other hand, those who are independent thinkers should be allowed to choose whatever professional assistance they wish if they feel they will derive benefit from it, without being made to feel guilty or peculiar just because it is different.

I have surveyed the opinion of some well qualified medical scientists who graduated from one of the best medical school in the United States of America about what they think of an alternative medicine like herbalism. Their reply was not different from the reply of their colleagues who went to recognised allopathic medical colleges in developed countries. They replied that "we think each group, whether it is chiropractic, osteopathic, naturopathic, acupuncture, homeopathic and traditional medicine has something to contribute." It is their opinion that "no one of us has the only right method; a patient should be entitled to help from all methods according to his needs."

UNDERSTANDING AND CO-OPERATION ARE NEEDED

To sum up what ought to be the attitude of all the healing professions:-

The physician does not cure, be he a natural, medical, or drug-and-surgical practitioner. Activation of the patients' inherent powers of recovery by natural means can best restore normal functions.

Traditional medical practitioners, in the eyes of the law and the courts, are also practicing medicine, and can therefore be classified as medical doctors, practitioners and physicians regardless of the branch, system and method they are licensed to practice.

Therefore I think all medical practitioners should pool their intellectual efforts and financial resources and co-operate enthusiastically in an educational and legislative programme for the best health care for the greatest number, with equal rights and liberties of all lay individuals and groups of adult age and sound mind.

In my view, it is more important for people to get well and stay well than to quibble over who is best qualified to give help. The time is ripe that every shred of information needed to ensure health for mankind by the year 2000 is obtained, no matter whoever contributes that help, or where it comes from, as long as it is not harmful. The choice of all branches of healing, and of any substances, whether vitamins, herbs or food, should lie in the hands of the people as their God-given right to treat their own bodies as they see it fit.

It is my firm belief that all systems of medicine are complementary and adjunctive one to the other, and that one day there will be one medicine and one medicine only in order to give total health for all by the year 2000.

The recent acceptance as official policy by the World Health Organization (WHO) of the need to mobilize traditional systems of medicine in developing countries in addition to the practice of modern medicine in those countries in order to ensure "total health-care delivery" is a firm pointer that the trend in official international circles is now obviously in that direction.

Once more I thank the organizers of the Long Island Philosophical Society for inviting me to present this paper. I thank the audience for their patience.

God Bless you all.

REFERENCES

1. David Landy. *Culture, Disease and Healing.* 1977.
2. *Proceedings of the International Symposium on "Traditional Medical Therapy,"* 1973.
3. Chief Ajani Olujare. *African Herbs and Plants.* 1963.
4. *African Medicinal Plants.* 1979.
5. Malcolm Hulke. *The Encyclopedia of Alternative Medicine and Self Help.* 1978.
6. Abayomi Sofowora. "African Medicinal Plants." *Proceedings of the Conference.* 1979.
7. *Daily Times,* February. 18th, 1987. "Lembo Wants Traditional Doctor Defined."
8. Dr. S. Olude. *Mediconsult.* No. 31, February-March, 1986.
9. *Clinical Pharmacy and Herbal Medicine,* Vol. 2, No. 5, September/October, 1986.
10. *Clinical Pharmacy and Herbal Medicine,* Vol. 2, 1986.
11. "Nigerian Medicinal Plants," *Zac Ogbile,* 21st-25th July, 1985.
12. Z.O. Gbile, M.O. Soladoye and S.K. Adesina. *Plants in Traditional Medicine in West Africa.* 1985.
13. Ayo Baiyelo. *Towards Blue Print of Education in Trado- Science.* September, 1986.
14. Sofowora. *Proceeding of a Workshop on Medicinal Plants Research in Nigeria.* 1986.

NOTES ON THE CONTRIBUTORS

HUSSAIN O.T. AJALA is a Doctor of Chiropractic and a Research Fellow II at the National Institute for Medical Research in Lagos, Nigeria. He is a member of the Nigerian Council of Traditional Medicine Practitioners and the Secretary of the Nigeria Alternative Medical Association.

MICHAEL D. BAYLES is professor of philosophy at Florida State University. He has been a fellow at Harvard Law School, the Hastings Center, and the National Humanities Center. He has also been director of the Westminster Institute for Ethics and Human Values in London, Canada. Among his published books are *Professional Ethics* (2nd edition, 1988), *Principles of Law* (1987), and *Reproductive Ethics* (1984).

MARGARET P. BENNER, R.N., Ph.D., is an Assistant Professor in the Department of Nursing Science, College of Nursing, University of Delaware. Her doctoral degree in Philosophy of Education with a focus on Nursing Ethics. She is a member of the Research Committee of Delaware Hospice, Inc.

MICHAEL BRANNIGAN is currently Associate Professor of Philosophy and Religion at Mercy College in Dobbs Ferry, New York. He received his Ph.D. in Philosophy and M.A. in Religious Studies from the University of Louvain in Belgium. He has published works in both medical ethics and Oriental philosophy.

JANE KREPLICK BRODY received her Ph.D. in 1987 from Adelphi University for a dissertation on ethical decision making in nursing. She was formerly an instructor at Villanova University College of Nursing, and a staff nurse at Vanderbilt University Hospital. She is presently an assistant professor at Molloy College on Long Island.

SALVATOR CANNAVO, Ph.D., is Professor Emeritus of Philosophy at Brooklyn College (CUNY). He is the author of *Nomic Inference* (Problems in the Logic of Scientific Inquiry) and of journal articles in the

219

philosophy of science, aesthetics, and analytical philosophy.

BEVERLEE ANN COX, Ph.D., is Professor and former Dean of the Faculty of Nursing of the University of Western Ontario. She teaches in the areas of psychiatry and mental health practice; biomedical ethics; and theories of psychopathology. She has done research in these areas and has presented her findings at conferences in Canada, the United States and Europe in recent years. Her current research interests, in addition to the above, include proposed studies of suicidal behavior among the elderly; community mental health resources; and dysfunctional communication patterns in families.

WILLIAM F. FINN, M.D., is honorary gynecologist at the North Shore University Hospital, and chairman of the ethics committee of the Episcopal Health Services. He is presently a doctoral candidate in philosophy at the Graduate Center of the City University of New York.

BETH FURLONG, R.N.C., M.S., M.A., has taught Community Health Nursing at Creighton University for the past sixteen years. A member of the Nebraska Nurses Association, she has been active in wellness-related activities for the past ten years. She presently serves as co-chair of Creighton's Wellness Council and is a member of the Board of Directors of the Wellness council for the Midlands.

RICHARD E. HART received his Ph.D. from SUNY-Stony Brook. He is currently Assistant Professor of Philosophy at Bloomfield College, New Jersey. He has published articles and reviews in applied ethics, natural law theory, philosophy and literature, the teaching of philosophy and on such figures as Buber, Socrates, and Brecht. His doctoral research concerned the relation between metaphysics and literary theory. Presently, he teaches courses in interdisciplinary humanities, logic, and a variety of applied ethics areas.

EUGENE KELLY, Ph.D., has been the chairman of the Long Island Philosophical Society since 1982. He is the author of a book and several articles on the philosophy of Max Scheler, and has published work on Continental aesthetics and American philosophy. He is the co-author of several textbooks, including *An Invitation to Philosophy* (Prometheus, 1981). He teaches at the New York Institute of Technology.

CHRISTOPHER P. MOONEY is currently Professor and Chairman in the Philosophy Department of Nassau Community College. He received his B.A . from Columbia University, and his M.A. and Ph.D. from Fordham University. He has published widely on the history and practice of philosophy. One of is major areas of interest is the interface between legal and ethical prohibitions.

DOROTHY H. MOSER, R.N., M.Ed., is an Associate Professor in the Department of Nursing Science, College of Nursing, University of Delaware. She has been a Trustee of Delaware Hospice, Inc. since its inception and teaches a hospice nursing course. She also had a sabbatical fellowship for a clinical practicum in Medical Ethics at the University of Tennessee, Center for Health Sciences in the Program on Human Values and Ethics.

JAMES MUYSKENS is Acting Provost at Hunter College of the City University of New York. He is the author of *Moral Problems in Nursing: A Philosophical Investigation* and *The Sufficiency of Hope* as well as numerous articles in bioethics and the philosophy of religion. He holds a Ph.D. in philosophy from the University of Michigan and an M.Div. from Princeton Theological Seminary.

LEON PEARL received his Ph.D. in philosophy from New York University in 1957. He has been a Professor at Hofstra University since 1960. His publications include *Descartes* (Twayne, 1977), *Four Philosophical Problems* (Harper and Row, 1963), and articles in *Mind* and *Philosophy and Phenomenological*

Research. He is a practicing attorney in New York State.

LOUIS SPORTELLI is a Doctor of Chiropractic, with a practice in Palmerton, Pennsylvania. The author of many articles in the American Chiropractic Association's *Journal of Chiropractic* and elsewhere, he has also made substantive contributions to chiropractic technique. He was named Pennsylvania Chiropractor of the Year in 1975, and has made numerous appearances on radio and television as a spokesman for chiropractic.

JOHN GREENFELDER SULLIVAN holds two earned doctorates: one in ecclesiastical law from the Lateran University in Rome and another in philosophy from the University of North Carolina at Chapel Hill. Formerly the Assistant Chancellor of the Roman Catholic diocese of Rhode Island, he is presently Maude Sharpe Powell Professor of Philosophy at Elon College. He serves on the Board of Trustees of the Traditional Acupuncture Institute in Columbia, Maryland.